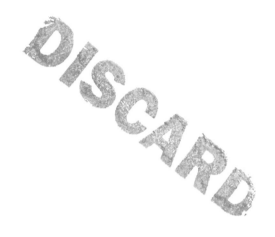

Creativity and Mental Illness

Creativity and Mental Illness

The Mad Genius in Question

Simon Kyaga
Karolinska Institutet, Sweden

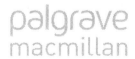

First published 2015 by
PALGRAVE MACMILLAN

Palgrave Macmillan in the UK is an imprint of Macmillan Publishers Limited, registered in England, company number 785998, of Houndmills, Basingstoke, Hampshire RG21 6XS.

Palgrave Macmillan in the US is a division of St Martin's Press LLC, 175 Fifth Avenue, New York, NY 10010.

Palgrave Macmillan is the global academic imprint of the above companies and has companies and representatives throughout the world.

Palgrave® and Macmillan® are registered trademarks in the United States, the United Kingdom, Europe and other countries.

ISBN 978–1–137–34580–6

This book is printed on paper suitable for recycling and made from fully managed and sustained forest sources. Logging, pulping and manufacturing processes are expected to conform to the environmental regulations of the country of origin.

A catalogue record for this book is available from the British Library.

Library of Congress Cataloging-in-Publication Data
Kyaga, Simon, 1976–
Creativity and mental illness : the mad genius in question / Simon Kyaga.
pages cm
ISBN 978–1–137–34580–6 (hardback)
1. Genius and mental illness.   2. Creative ability—Psychological aspects.
I. Title.
BF423.K93   2015
153.3'5—dc23   2014023285

Typeset by MPS Limited, Chennai, India.

Transferred to Digital Printing in 2015

Contents

Tables, Figures and Boxes

Tables

Figures

Boxes

Preface

This book is the result of a common observation among clinicians in psychiatry, that some of those suffering mental illness are also capable of remarkable achievements (Becker, 1978, p 658). One of the first patients I had the opportunity to meet in this context was diagnosed with bipolar I disorder. He was in a terrible state, struck by symptoms of depression with melancholic features. His whole person displayed a complete absence of energy; I found myself incapable of imagining him as a great entrepreneur. However, on my second visit to him, together with his wife, I was told that just a few months earlier, in the summer, he had celebrated his fiftieth birthday on an island in the Swedish archipelago, with hundreds of guests participating. In his usual abundance of energy, his wife said, he had been able to convince a Swedish fighter pilot to fly over the island in a show much appreciated by the people below. As we sat in the small room at the hospital, it was winter and there was snow falling outside the window. I looked at him and realized that *this* was bipolar disorder.

Simon Kyaga
Karolinska Institutet

Acknowledgements

Cover illustration by Dennis Eriksson, Copyright 2014, with permission from Woo.

Figure 2.2 is reprinted from *Journal of Affective Disorders*, 100, Hagop S. Akiskal, Kareen K., 'In search of Aristotle: Temperament, human nature, melancholia, creativity and eminence', 1–6, Copyright 2007, with permission from Elsevier.

Figure 4.1 is reprinted from the *Journal of Creative Behavior*, 43(2), Kaufman, J.C., Cole, J.C. and Baer, J., 'The Construct of Creativity: Structural Model for Self-Reported Creativity Ratings', 119–34, Copyright 2009, with permission from John Wiley and Sons.

Figure 4.2 is reprinted from the *Personality and Social Psychology Review*, 2(4), Gregory J. Feist, 'A Meta-Analysis of Personality in Scientific and Artistic Creativity', 290–309, Copyright 1998, with permission from Sage.

Abbreviations

16-PF	Sixteen personality factor questionnaire
5-HT	Serotonin
BWAS	Barron–Welsh art scale
CAQ	Creativity achievement questionnaire
CAT	Computerized axial tomography (CT scanning)
CAT	Consensual assessment technique
COMT	Catechol-O-methyltransferase
DRD2	Dopamine receptor D2
DZ	Dizygotic
EEG	Electroencephalography
EPQ	Eysenck personality questionnaire
FFM	Five factor model of personality
fMRI	Functional magnetic resonance imaging
IPAR	Institute of Personality Assessment and Research
MRI	Magnetic resonance imaging
MZ	Monozygotic
NEO PI-R	NEO personality inventory – revised
PET	Positron emission tomography
PFC	Prefrontal cortex
RAT	Remote associates test
RIBS	Runco ideational behavior scale
rTMS	Repetitive transcranial magnetic stimulation
SOI	Guilford's structure of intellect
SPECT	Single photon emission computed tomography
TEMPS-A	Temperament evaluation of the Memphis, Pisa, Paris, and San Diego autoquestionnaire
TTCT	Torrance tests of creative thinking

1
Introduction

We have many books and articles on great men, their genius, their heredity, their insanity, their precocity, their versatility and the like, but, whether these are collections of anecdotes such as Professor Lombroso's or scientific investigations such as Dr Galton's, they are lacking in exact and quantitative deductions. Admitting that genius is hereditary, or, what is more doubtful, that it is likely to be associated with insanity, we have only the 'yes' or 'no' as our answer. But this is only the beginning of science. Science asks how much? We can only answer when we have an objective series of observations, sufficient to eliminate chance errors.

James Cattell in 'A Statistical Study
of Eminent Men' (1903)

Is there really a thin line between madness and genius? While many of us inherently are inclined to believe so, history is full of ideas that science has disproven. The aim of this book is to discuss the present state of knowledge on the alleged association between creativity and mental illness: if there is a true association, and if so, how this association is manifested.

The mad genius link

Comments on the mad genius link have been made almost as long as Western society itself. Often referred is Aristotle's (384–322 BC) question put in *Problemata XXX*, written by his pupil Theophrast (371–287 BC), 'Why is it that all those who have become eminent in philosophy, politics, poetry, or the arts are clearly melancholics and some of them

1

to such an extent as to be affected by diseases caused by the black bile?' (Aristotle, 1984). This quote was later modified by Seneca the Younger (4 BC–AD 65) citing Aristotle to have said, 'No great genius has existed without a strain of madness' (Motto and Clark, 1992). Later times saw the poet John Dryden allude to this quote, arguing that, 'Great wits are sure to madness near ally'd; and thin partitions do their bounds divide' (Motto and Clark, 1992). A famous quote by the romantic poet Samuel Coleridge, was that his madness was, 'a madness, indeed celestial, and glowing from a divine mind' (Sanborn, 1886). The end of the ninteenth century also saw the birth of more scientifically inclined studies on the alleged association of creativity and mental illness. Of these, Cesare Lombroso's study had an enduring impact on public apprehension (1891). However, as can be found in the quote by James Cattell above (1903), Lombroso fell into disrepute, and his work has since been considered as a mere collection of anecdotes.

Research in creativity has expanded considerably since then (Kaufman and Sternberg, 2010). Today a multitude of questions maintain the interest of an ever increasing number of researchers focused on different aspects of creativity. Creativity, as an object of study, is a multifaceted entity that by nature is translational. Thus, creativity is approached in a number of disciplines, such as psychology, sociology, pedagogy, history, economy and, more recently, by genetics and neuroscience (Kaufman and Sternberg, 2010). Nonetheless, the interest in the old question of the mad genius link has been upheld both within academia, and what is perhaps more uncommon for a scholarly field, within the public (Silvia and Kaufman, 2010).

This is maybe the reason why researchers who are otherwise stringent and subjected to rational thought, may sometimes be carried away when discussing the nature of creativity and psychopathology. The field is characterized by authors having taken completely contradictory positions arguing everything from mental illness having nothing to do with creativity to other authors arguing for it being deeply entwined. Many times these arguments are passionate and often less founded in empirical studies (Silvia and Kaufman, 2010).

Early empirical studies on creativity and mental illness

Lombroso's study of genius linked to madness was contemporary with other attempts to approach the question of genius with a burgeoning empirical approach. Francis Galton's *Hereditary Genius – An Inquiry into its Laws and Consequences* published in 1869 was a comprehensive attempt to investigate hereditary aspects of exceptional behaviour (1869). In *English Men of Science: Their nature and nurture* published in 1874 (1874), Galton concluded with a reference to Thomas Carlyle that, 'It is maintained by Helvetius and his set, that an infant of genius is quite the same as any other infant, only that certain surprisingly favourable influences accompany him through life ... I should as soon agree as with this other – that acorn might, by favourable or unfavourable influences of soil and climate, be nursed into a cabbage, or the cabbage-seed into an oak' (p. ix).

Thus, much of the early studies into genius were driven by the idea that certain inborn traits were associated with extraordinary gifts. However, in 1928 Wilhelm Lange-Eichbaum argued for a sociological perspective on the definition of genius. In an English shortened version of his vast *Genie – Irrsinn und Ruhm* published in 1931, he claims that, 'The one who is not yet called a genius is no genius' (Lange-Eichbaum and Paul, 1931, p. 67). Yet, he says, 'It cannot be a chance matter that among geniuses the healthy constitute a minority' (p. 125).

Rise of creativity research

Although there had been early attempts to characterize the creative process, it was Joy Paul Guilford who introduced creativity as an important field for psychological research. In his 1950s inaugural address to the American Psychological Association, Guilford characterized creativity as the most important resource available to human society (1950). He told that efforts to promote creativity would pay high dividends for society as a whole. Guilford also promoted the use of *psychometrics*, the measurement of creativity objectively, and argued for divergent thinking being at the heart of the creative process. Divergent thinking does not result in one right answer but rather in a number of possible solutions to an open-ended problem. Although Guilford's idea of divergent thinking as a common factor for creativity has been debated in recent research, his influence still carries weight in the field (Runco, 2010).

Contemporary studies on the mad genius link

Increasingly studies using sound methods have investigated the question of a link between genius and madness or more specifically creativity and psychopathology.

Nancy Andreasen, for example, demonstrated increased risk for affective disorders (depression, bipolar disorder) in general and for bipolar disorder in particular in 30 creative writers at the University of Iowa writers' workshop, compared to healthy controls (1987). Similarly, Kay Redfield Jamison found increased risk for affective disorders in 47 British writers (1989). Arnold Ludwig used reviews of biographies published in the *New York Times* book review between 1960 and 1990 as selection criteria, identifying 1005 eminent individuals (1992, 1995). Based on their biographies, he found an overrepresentation of bipolar disorder, schizophrenia-like psychosis and depression in the creative arts group.

The above studies are often cited in defence of the alleged association between creativity and mental illness. They have, however, been seriously criticized by some authors opposing the association between creativity and mental illness (Rothenberg, 1995). Judith Schlesinger goes as far as to call the whole association a *hoax* (2009, 2012). Schlesinger's main criticism is that the authors of these studies both selected study subjects, and in general themselves made the diagnoses without support in recognized diagnostic manuals. This would make the results open to both bias and difficulties in generalization. While part of Schlesinger's criticism is relevant and sound scepticism is always advised, there is a surprising neglect in Schlesinger's approach to discuss or even mention the other roughly hundred empirical studies addressing the association between creativity and psychopathology.

Some of these other studies have evaluated creativity in people with manifest psychopathology. Santosa et al. compared individuals with bipolar disorder, unipolar depression, healthy creative, and non-creative controls using the creative inventory Barron-Welsh Art Scale (BWAS) (2007). They found that people with bipolar disorder and healthy creative controls scored higher than those with unipolar depression and non-creative controls. Another study reported increased creativity in 40 American adults with bipolar disorder compared with healthy controls using the same instrument (Simeonova et al., 2005).

To avoid bias caused by the debilitating effects of mental illness, some studies have included relatives of those with psychiatric disorders. For example, Karlsson investigated 486 male relatives of people with schizophrenia born in Iceland between 1851 and 1940 (1970). Compared with the general population, the relatives were more often represented in a listing of prominent people. There was also a significant increase in those specifically successful in creative endeavours, although the number of people included were small.

Because most of earlier studies have relied on biographical data of eminent individuals or small cohorts of patients, we initiated a project using large scale population-based methods to investigate the association of

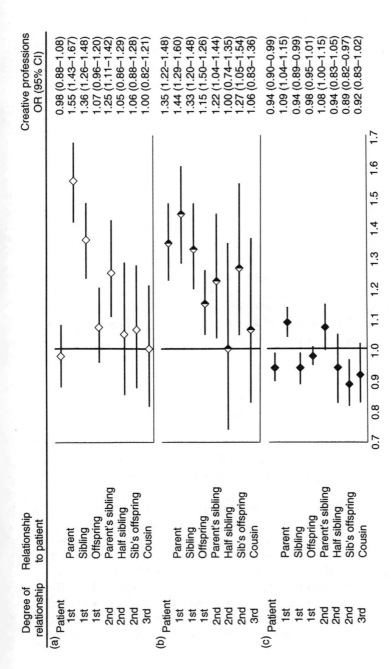

Figure 1.1 Study on ~300000 patients demonstrating an increased occurrence of creative professions in patients with bipolar disorder (A) and healthy relatives of patients with schizophrenia (B) and bipolar disorder compared to healthy controls.

Note: No associations were found for patients with unipolar depression (C) or their relatives. An odds ratio (OR) higher than 1 implies an increased occurrence, whereas lower than 1 implies a decreased occurrence. Creative professions were defined as artistic and scientific occupations.

Source: Kyaga et al., 2011.

creativity and psychopathology. In the first study ~300000 patients with schizophrenia, bipolar disorder and unipolar depression, and all of these patients' healthy relatives (first, second, third degree), were investigated with regards to their representation in creative professions (Kyaga et al., 2011). Creative professions were defined as artistic and scientific occupations. Results demonstrated a significant increase of creative professions in patients with bipolar disorder and relatives of patients with schizophrenia and bipolar disorder (Figure 1.1). No associations were found for patients with unipolar depression or their relatives. Common for schizophrenia and bipolar disorder is that they are psychotic disorders. Psychosis is a severe symptom consisting of an aberrant comprehension of reality (Box 1.1).

The results of the first study was later followed up in a larger set of ~1.2 million psychiatric patients and their relatives including most different psychiatric disorders (Kyaga et al., 2013). Results affirmed previous associations, but also suggested an association for relatives of patients with anorexia nervosa and possibly autism. Most other psychiatric diagnoses, such as unipolar depression, anxiety disorders and substance abuse were associated with a decrease in the likelihood of holding creative professions. However, authors were specifically affected with most psychiatric disorders and also suffered a ~50 per cent increase in the risk of committing suicide.

Box 1.1   History of psychiatric diagnoses

Research into the clinical manifestation (phenomenology) of psychiatric disorders has a long history. The word disorder is derived from the French word *désordre*, meaning disorder, disturbance or chaos. This deviance from norm is traditionally seen in relation to a statistical norm (e.g., population mean), cultural norm or the individual self.

Modern definitions of psychiatric disorder rests heavily on the work of Emil Kraepelin (1856–1926). In his *Compendium der Psychiatrie* published in 1883, he argues that psychiatry is a branch of medical science that should be investigated by observation and experimentation like other natural sciences. He proposed that by studying case histories and identifying specific disorders, the prognosis of specific mental illnesses could be made, after taking into account individual differences in personality. Kraepelin divided psychosis (then meaning severe psychiatric disorder) into two distinct forms, acknowledged as the Kraepelinian dichotomy: manic depression and dementia praecox. Manic depression corresponded to more contemporary definitions of recurrent major depression and bipolar disorder, while dementia praecox was later redefined by Eugen Bleuler (1857–1939) as Schizophrenia. The later was to stress that dementia praecox did not necessarily lead to mental decline, which was initially proposed by Kraepelin. For a description of the phenomenology of the most common psychiatric disorders, please refer to Box 1.2.

Classifications systems

Contemporary psychiatry uses one of two systems to classify psychiatric disorders. These are the *International Statistical Classification of Diseases and Related Health Problems* (ICD) or the *Diagnostic and Statistical Manual of Mental Disorders* (DSM). Both these systems have been continuously updated. The ICD, presently in its tenth version (ICD-10) is provided by the World Health Organization (WHO), which is a branch of the United Nations (2004). The main office is in Geneva, Switzerland. The first version headed by the WHO was published in 1948 (ICD-6), which was based on work, however, by the Frenchman Jaques Bertillon presented at the International Statistical Institute in 1893 (2010). The current ICD version was accepted in 1990 and consequently adopted by member countries during the following years. It is the internationally accepted standard for diagnosis of diseases and used for epidemiological and statistical purposes.

In parallel with the development of the ICD, the 1970s saw a growth of interest in refining psychiatric classification worldwide (1993). Several national psychiatric organizations developed specific criteria for classifications in order to improve diagnostic reliability. In particular, the American Psychiatric Association developed and disseminated its Third Revision of the Diagnostic and Statistical Manual of Mental Disorders (DSM-III-Tr) (American Psychiatric Association. Task Force on Nomenclature and Statistics. & American Psychiatric Association. Committee on Nomenclature and Statistics, 1980). This system incorporated operational criteria into its classification system, meaning that certain criteria were set up as an aid for the clinician to make diagnosis. The main reason for this was to improve reliability, which at the time had been seriously questioned for psychiatric diagnosis (Andreasen, 2007). The DSM is presently in its fifth edition, released in May 2013 (American Psychiatric Association & American Psychiatric Association. DSM-5 Task Force, 2013).

Box 1.2 Brief phenomenology of some major psychiatric diagnoses

Schizophrenia

Aberrations in one or more of the following five areas: delusions, hallucinations, disorganized thinking, grossly disorganized motor behaviour, and negative symptoms (diminished emotional expression and avolition) (American Psychiatric Association & American Psychiatric Association. DSM-5 Task Force, 2013).

Bipolar disorder

Presence of intermittent manic or hypomanic (less severe) episodes; a period in which there is an abnormally, elevated, expansive, or irritable mood and increased activity or energy that is present for most of the day, nearly every day, for a period of at least 1 week (4 days for hypomania) (American Psychiatric Association & American Psychiatric Association. DSM-5 Task Force, 2013). *Bipolar I disorder* refers to the presence of manic episodes, whereas hypomanic episodes define *bipolar II disorder*. In general a patient diagnosed with bipolar disorder also suffers recurrent depressive episodes. Within this group of disorders, the DSM-5 also defines *cyclothymic disorder* as fluctuating mood disturbance with hypomanic symptoms that are of insufficient number, severity, pervasiveness, or duration to meet criteria of a hypomanic episode, and the depressive symptoms similarly insufficient to meet criteria for a major depressive episode.

Unipolar depression (major depressive disorder)

Presence of a period of minimum 2 weeks during which there is either depressed mood or the loss of interest in virtually all activities (American Psychiatric Association & American Psychiatric Association. DSM-5 Task Force, 2013).

Anxiety disorders

Anxiety disorders differ from general fear or anxiety by being disproportionate or continuing beyond developmentally applicable periods. The different anxiety disorders are characterized by the types of objects or situations that prompt fear; specific phobias, social phobia, panic disorder etc. (American Psychiatric Association & American Psychiatric Association. DSM-5 Task Force, 2013).

Substance abuse disorders

A set of disorders characterized by impaired control, social impairment, risky use (physically and psychologically hazardous) and pharmacological criteria (tolerance and withdrawal symptoms) (American Psychiatric Association & American Psychiatric Association. DSM-5 Task Force, 2013).

Autism spectrum disorders

Persistent deficiency in social interaction and repetitive patterns of behaviour or interests, with symptoms present from early childhood impairing everyday function (American Psychiatric Association & American Psychiatric Association. DSM-5 Task Force, 2013).

ADHD

A persistent history from childhood of inattention and/or hyperactivity-impulsivity that hinders functioning or development (American Psychiatric Association & American Psychiatric Association. DSM-5 Task Force, 2013).

Intellectual disability

Discrepancies in general mental abilities and impairment in everyday functioning, compared to an individual's age-, gender-, and socioculturally matched peers (American Psychiatric Association & American Psychiatric Association. DSM-5 Task Force, 2013).

Anorexia nervosa

Main features are food restriction, intense fear of gaining weight or persistent behaviour interfering with weight gain, and a disturbance in self-perceived weight or shape (American Psychiatric Association & American Psychiatric Association. DSM-5 Task Force, 2013).

Box 1.3 Psychosis

Psychosis in its contemporary meaning implies impaired reality-testing ability (Stern, 2008). The most important features are hallucinations and delusions. Psychosis is not a mental disorder, but a symptom present across different psychiatric disorders.

The term was established in 1845 by Feuchtersleben for all mental disorders since he believed that these were 'diseases of the personality' resulting from an interplay between body and mind (Beer, 1996). The purpose was to refrain from using other then-present descriptions of mental disorders, such as 'Geisteskrankheiten' and 'Seelenstörungen' placing too much emphasis on the mind. The initial meaning of psychosis was thus simply mental disorder. This definition was upheld by Kraepelin in the first edition of his textbook published in 1896, but successively narrowed and finally in the ninth edition, Kraepelin designated dementia praecox (renamed schizophrenia by Eugen Bleuler) and manic-depressive insanity as the only two true psychotic disorders.

This idea continues in today's nosological division between schizophrenia and bipolar disorder (American Psychiatric Association & American Psychiatric Association. DSM-5 Task Force, 2013), although the interpretation of psychosis has now changed into being a symptom of compromised reality-testing. Still, psychosis in this contemporary meaning is also a defining clinical feature of schizophrenia and often present in severe bipolar disorder.

Biological aspects of creativity

One of the most fascinating developments in creativity research concerns new findings on the biology of creativity (Runco, 2007a). This has partly been made possible by the introduction of modern neuroimaging techniques, such as magnetic resonance imaging (MRI), functional MRI (fMRI) and positron emission tomography (PET) (Box 1.4). These methods provide possibilities to investigate both structure and function of the brain in living humans.

Changes in hemispheric asymmetries of the brain have long been proposed as an important mechanism underlying increased creativity in certain individuals. In humans the left hemisphere is generally dominant. While ideas of hemispheric asymmetries have a long history in psychiatry, it was Roger Sperry's investigations of split-brain patients in the 1970s that truly fuelled interest in hemispheric asymmetries underlying creativity (Sperry, 1964).

These patients had been operated for severe epilepsy, with a disconnecting of the two hemispheres through the destruction of the corpus callosum, a wide, flat bundle of neural fibres connecting the cerebral hemispheres. This structure normally functions as the main communication channel for the two hemispheres. The purpose for the operation was to inhibit the spread or *generalization* of epileptic activity over the brain. However, the operation also made it possible to investigate the separate functions of the two hemispheres. It was concluded that the right hemisphere specializes in parallel and global processes, whereas the left hemisphere mainly uses sequential and analytical processes (Katz, 1997; Sperry, 1964).

More recent studies using fMRI have later provided evidence that the right hemisphere is specifically implicated in creativity. For instance, one study using fMRI saw activations in the right prefrontal cortex (PFC) (i.e., the front of the frontal cortex) in a creative story generation task (Howard-Jones et al., 2005). The PFC has received much interest from researchers in creativity (Gonen-Yaacovi et al., 2013; Runco, 2007a). It is considered responsible for higher mental functions, such as attention, working memory, and cognitive flexibility (Dietrich, 2004; Runco, 2007a).

Interestingly, even direct manipulations of brain activity have been associated with changes in creative and associated behaviours. By using repetitive transcranial magnetic stimulation (rTMS) Synder et al. created temporary 'lesions' of the fronto-temporal lobes in 11 healthy individuals (2003). Following this manipulation research subjects made drawings considered by a committee as more life-like, flamboyant, and complex.

Another field that has received increasing amount of attention in creativity research is the search for specific genes underlying creativity (Runco, 2007a). As previously mentioned, Galton was clearly of the impression that certain heritable characteristics were associated with genius (1869, 1874). This idea was later affirmed in Cox's comprehensive study from 1926 on 301 of the most eminent men and women of history (Cox et al., 1926). The first comparison between twins with regards to creative interests was made by Carter in 1932, who found the genetic component to explain ~60 per cent of the variance for vocational interest in artistic occupations (1932). Another study estimated the heritability for interest in science to ~39 per cent, however, for divergent thinking the heritability was only ~20 per cent (Nichols, 1978).

The first molecular gene study of creativity was conducted by Reuter et al. in 2006 demonstrating a significant association between dopamine D2 receptor gene and a serotonergic gene, TPH1, in a sample of 92 healthy subjects (Reuter et al., 2006). Some of these findings were partly replicated in a later study (M. Murphy et al., 2013; Runco et al., 2011).

With the development of research in creativity, beneficial health effects of creativity have been increasingly stressed (Runco, 2007a). Thus, many studies argue that creative activities can be stress reducing. For instance, one study of musicians found high levels of creativity to be associated with low levels of stress (Nicol and Long, 1996). Other authors have argued for creativity as a capacity to adapt, which would have beneficial effects for coping in life (Runco, 2007a). In fact writing about emotional experiences has been associated with both biological increases in immune efficiency and significant reductions in reported distress (Pennebaker, 1997).

Box 1.4   Neuroimaging and related methods

Neuroimaging refers to the use of different techniques to image the brain's structure (e.g., CAT and MRI) or function (e.g., SPECT, PET, fMRI).

Allan McLeod Cormack and Godfrey Newbold Hounsfield introduced computerized axial tomography (CAT or CT scanning) in the 1970s allowing for detailed anatomical images of the brain. This invention was rewarded with the 1979 Nobel Prize for medicine. Following the introduction of CAT, the development of radioactive ligands resulted in SPECT and PET. These later methods allowed for the investigation of both cerebral blood flow and presence of different brain receptors. Concurrently MRI was developed by Peter Mansfield and Paul Lauterbur, who were awarded the 2003 Nobel Prize for medicine. MRI was later developed into fMRI measuring cerebral blood flow changes. MRI and fMRI has lately become more common than for example PET in the brain-mapping field owing to low invasiveness, absence of radiation exposure, and wide availability.

rTMS

Transcranial magnetic stimulation (TMS) is a non-invasive method to depolarize or hyperpolarize neurons (nerve cells) in the brain. It uses electromagnetic fields to induce weak electric activity. A variant of TMS, repetitive transcranial magnetic stimulation (rTMS) produces longer-lasting effects continuing after the initial stimulation. rTMS has been tested in the treatment of several neurological and psychiatric disorders.

What this book is about

This book is about the alleged association between creativity and mental illness. The aim is not to provide a grand theory, but rather a broad overview of current knowledge based on empirical observations, while also commenting on the vast literature related to the topic. The intention is to use an accessible language primarily aimed at students and scholars in creativity, innovation, psychology, clinical psychology and medicine, as well as residents and consultants in psychiatry. In addition, this book will most likely be suited for a broader audience outside of academia, who want to know more about the ancient idea of the mad genius.

The field of creativity research is translational and growing quickly. While it attempts to make a broad review on the association between creativity and mental illness, this book specifically focuses on recent advances in the *biology of creativity*.

The putative association between creativity and psychopathology, interesting in its own sense, also has implications for the care of patients with psychiatric disorders. While the literature is clearly in favour for treatment of patients with severe psychiatric disorders, the potential association between creativity and mental illness stresses the importance of listening to the experiences of each *individual* patient. Evidence-based medicine is defined as 'the conscientious, explicit, and judicious use of current best evidence in making decisions about the care of *individual* patients' (Sackett et al., 1996). Thus, it is vital to incorporate results from large clinical trials with individual information gathered by the clinician for the benefit of each patient.

2
The History of the Mad Genius

Why is it that all those who have become eminent in philosophy or politics or poetry or the arts are clearly melancholics and some of them to such an extent as to be affected by diseases caused by black bile?
Aristotle in *Problemata XXX* (1984)

Introduction

Many studies on the alleged association between creativity and mental illness choose to reference historical quotes by famous thinkers as the one by Aristotle above. It is congenital to ask why modern scientists should feel obliged to reference more than 2000-year-old philosophers in their contemporary research. The fact of the matter is that the question of genius and madness is as much a scholarly field as an ongoing argument with real implications for both creative individuals, especially artists, and psychiatric patients. Referencing prominent historical individuals thus serves an important part of providing credibility to the proposed association between genius and madness. However, as poignantly put by George Becker, the leading scholar on the historical background of the mad genius link, while the anecdotes affirming an association for genius with *divine madness* have been historically abundant, the idea of creativity being associated with *clinical madness* seems to be a modern invention not predating the 1830s (Becker, 2000, 2014).

The present chapter serves to trace the origins of the mad genius link and thereby providing a historical context for more modern studies on creativity and psychopathology. There has been a recent surge of scientific interest in the alleged association of creativity and mental illness. This chapter argues that one reason for this is the advent of a distinctly biological and genetic orientation in the etiology of psychiatric disorders.

Socrates' demon

The first commentaries on the link between psychopathology and creative achievement were made by the ancient Greeks. These commentaries have often been adhered to when contemporary proponents of the mad genius link have argued their cause. However, central to the ancient idea of madness was to make a clear distinction between divine and human madness (Becker, 2000, 2014). Thus, Socrates' call on his demon was a way to ask for divine inspiration, rather than subjecting to madness. In line with this view, poets, priests, philosophers and sages were able to reflect the gods through the intervention of their demons. The creator was void of any talent, while the demonic intervention filled the poet and alike with a divine inspiration reflecting the gods. This inspiration was only attainable during certain mental states, such as in sleep or when affected by illness or possession (Rosen, 1980). Clearly demarcated from human madness, the divine madness was seen as a virtue, a state of mind that was strived for (Plato, 2005).

While Plato commented on the association between creative achievement and psychopathology (Plato, 2005), more often a quote by Aristotle is used as a starting point for historical excursions into the mad genius link. He asks (Akiskal and Akiskal, 2007; Aristotle, 1984), 'Why is it that all those who have become eminent in philosophy or politics or poetry or the arts are clearly melancholics and some of them to such an extent as to be affected by diseases caused by black bile?'. These wordings were later modified by Seneca the Younger (c. 4 BC–AD 65), who choose to finish his treatise *De Tranquillitate Animi* with a reference to the previous quote by Aristotle: 'Nullum magnum ingeniurn sine mixtura dementiaefuií (no great genius has existed without a strain of madness)', thus introducing a conflicting element with Stoic thought (Motto and Clark, 1992). A similar paradox was provided by Plato in *Phaedrus* compared to his other writings, where he otherwise argued for *wisdom* as the foremost of virtues (Plato, 2005).

Aristotle's original reference to eminence and melancholia was derived from the then prevailing *humoral theory*, closely associated with Hippocrates (Becker, 2014). This theory argued that disease was the consequence of an imbalance in the four basic fluids (humours): blood, black bile, yellow bile and phlegm (Adams, 1849). Each of these humours consisted of certain elementary qualities, such as heat, cold, dryness, and moistness. When these humours were balanced, the individual was considered healthy. But, when external or internal influences caused an excess or lack of any of these humours, disease was the result. Important in the humoral theory was the idea that certain human temperaments were linked to the composition of these humours. Thus, a dominance of blood resulted in a sanguine personality, whereas phlegm resulted in phlegmatic personality, yellow bile in choleric personality, and black bile in melancholic personality.

Hippocrates arguably also made the first clinical observation of melancholia (Adams, 1849; Akiskal and Akiskal, 2007): 'A woman of Thasos ... as a result of justified grief became morose, and although she did not take to her bed, she suffered from insomnia, loss of appetite ... she complained of fears and talked much; she showed despondency and ... talked at random and used foul language... many intense and continuous pains ... she leapt up and could not be restrained ...'.

This clinical observation has been considered as a clear case of bipolar disorder by contemporary researchers (Akiskal and Akiskal, 2007). However, Aristotle's original quote cannot be taken as a general account that bipolar disorder is associated with achievement, but rather that the melancholic temperament is the well for this association. Depending on the specific combination of humours, an individual with these traits was suggested either sane or psychiatrically affected (Wittkower and Wittkower, 2007). In fact, this view is coherent with recent theory in psychiatric phenomenology, where one considers a bipolar spectrum of traits

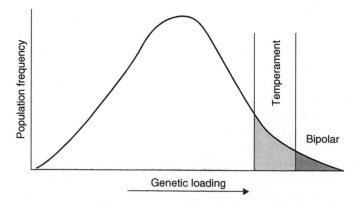

Figure 2.1   Bipolar spectrum.
Source: Akiskal and Akiskal, 2007, with permission from Elsevier.

seen on a scale ranging from severe bipolar disorder through less severe and on to affective temperaments, with the more severe cases increasingly established through genetic loading (Figure 2.1). Some argue that by linking melancholia and frenzy at the temperamental level, Aristotle may have been the first to describe this bipolar spectrum (Pies, 2007).

The Renaissance's imitatio-ideal

In Roman times and during the Middle Ages, less attention was dedicated to creative individuals (Becker, 2014); however, the Renaissance brought back a strong interest in persons with exceptional creative abilities. This renewed interest also incorporated those individuals with skills in sculpturing and painting, areas previously devalued by the Greeks owing to their dislike for manual work. Together with the exceptional poets and philosophers, the sculptors and painters were now considered as *genios*. However, quite different from modern times emphasizing originality, the Renaissance stressed the ability to *imitate* established masters and nature. Thus, more innovative creators at that time such as da Vinci and Vasari were not the rule but rather an exception (Zilsel, 1926).

Analogous to the Ancients' view, the Renaissance *genio* was often considered in terms of melancholia or *pazzia* (Becker, 2014). The separation between temperament and clinical insanity was still forcefully upheld. Ficinio, who helped disseminate the Aristotelian view during the Renaissance, regarded the melancholic temperament as a gift akin to Plato's divine madness clearly demarcated from human madness (Plato, 2005). Qualities associated with the melancholic temperament were eccentricity, sensitivity, moodiness and, to some extent, solitariness. During the sixteenth century these traits became greatly in vogue among artists (Wittkower and Wittkower, 2007). However, the fad was soon turned into a subject of criticism. As a consequence of the increasing criticism at the end of the sixteenth century, the seventeenth century witnessed a new ideal for the artist: the conforming gentleman artist merging with the social elites (Becker, 2014). It was the birth of the rational artist.

The rational artist

The Enlightenment introduced a new definition of genius. Considerably different from the Renaissance *imitatio-ideal*, the Enlightenment's genius was seen as someone who displayed ground-breaking *novelty and originality* (Lange-Eichbaum and Paul, 1931; Tonelli, 1973; Zilsel, 1926). The emphasis was now on rational thought, and the genius was seen as someone who could wisely balance mental forces into harmony. True genius was, according to Gerard (1774), the consequence of a synthesis of a) imagination, b) judgement, c) sense, and d) memory. While the creativity was born out of an active imagination, this imagination had to be tempered and 'subjected to established laws' (Becker, 2014; Gerard, 1774).

Thus, ideas on genius during the Enlightenment accepted sub rational components reflected in creative imagination, yet established judgement, or reason, as an important counterbalance to this faculty. This emphasis on rational judgement made it essentially impossible to accept *madness* – clinical or divine – as concurrent with genius (Becker, 2014).

The Romantic genius

A revolt against natural laws

The emphasis on rationality was, however, soon to be criticized; the late eighteenth and early nineteenth centuries witnessed a return of the artist and genius subjected to *unrestricted imagination and inspiration* (Becker, 2014). The Romantic's reaction to the mechanical stance of the Enlightenment was forceful. Inspired by a science influenced by new discoveries in chemistry and electricity, the Romantics saw the universe as a mysterious dwelling of oscillations, growth and organic change. Back was the divinely inspired genius, who in an enthusiastic spirit struggled for a reckless quest of truth, beauty and knowledge.

A historical necessity

Becker argues that it is also critically important to consider this dramatic change from rational to emotional in light of concurrent historic events leaving the Romantic poets and men of letters in a precarious state of existence (2014). The eighteenth century, as has been previously argued, had seen the making of a new form of *genius*, characterized by *novelty and originality*. Most of these individuals were deprived of wealth or privileged status, and consequently tended to challenge existing hierarchical order (Becker, 2014). D'Alembert, who contended a view held by many of the men of letters during the Enlightenment, saw three aspects separating people: *birth*, *wealth* and *intelligence*; however, only intelligence was argued to be worthy of true admiration (Becker, 2014).

The period following Napoleon's defeat, however, meant that these revolutionary ideas lost strength and that the potential of instituting intelligence as the principle for the ranking of men received a serious set-back. In all, the late eighteenth and early nineteenth centuries provided men of letters with a rather ungratifying position (Graña, 1964). The ensuing loss of influence meant that the aspiring intelligentsia lost their platform in society. It was in this political vacuum, that these artists and men of letters turned to the ancient idea of the genius as possessed by mad demons (Becker, 2000).

The making of a new genius

The idea that divine madness could distinguish the extraordinary individual provided artists and men of letters with a mystical aura separating them from ordinary individuals. It made them heirs in a long line of exceptional individuals emanating in antiquity, and provided them with privileges historically granted only to the prophets. Thus, the man of genius was permitted to speak freely in an otherwise dangerous way. In addition, the idea of succumbing to mania paralleled the Romantic notion of possession and suffering. For the Romantics, *imagination* was at the heart of the creative process, and any attempt to temper imagination by rationality would only obstruct its potential (Becker, 2014; Nordau, 1892/1993).

A dangerous strategy

The emphasis on imagination over rationality served as the main reason to free the Romantics from intellectual independence (Becker, 2014). As a consequence, however, they were also increasingly distanced from the mental qualities primarily associated with sanity. This provided an opening for the emergence of the idea of genius and clinical madness. Trapped by their own logic, the Romantics began to see madness as inescapable (Becker, 2014). Although many references were made to *divine* madness, increasingly authors also submitted to fears of genuine clinical insanity. Coleridge (quoted in Sanborn, 1886), for example, suggested that: 'The reason may resist for a long time ... but too often, at length, it yields for a moment, and the man is mad forever ... I think it was Bishop Butler who said that he was all his life struggling against the devilish suggestions on his senses, which would have maddened him if he had relaxed the stern wakefulness of his reason for a single moment.'

The growth of the medico-psychiatric field

The increasing fear of clinical madness among the Romantics was, however, not possible without the concomitant rise in psychology and the medical-psychiatric profession. During the eighteenth and nineteenth centuries, a school of thought was established known as faculty psychology (Boring, 1950). The ideas of this school was based on Aristotelian views of mind and creativity, recognizing distinct mental faculties that to some extent were open to enhancement through exercise (Becker, 2014). Reid, for example, argued 24 mental faculties recognizing, e.g., perception, judgement and moral taste, as distinct entities (Boring, 1950). While Reid and others acknowledged that these faculties could be improved through training, they also recognized that faculties were decidedly rooted in native disposition. The latter belief was highly congruent with the emergence of the genius ideal and its Romantic reformulation. Further to this, faculty psychology argued that over-stimulation of any faculty of mind was incompatible with health and sanity (Sully, 1884), a view highly concomitant with the Romantics' view that the genius's dependence on an unrestrained imagination constituted madness.

From the middle of the nineteenth century, the rise of the psychiatric field initiated a medical approach to the question of genius and madness. The first examination of genius from a medical standpoint was instigated by Lélut in 1836, who claimed that Socrates' habit of taking inspiration from the voice of a supernatural agent was confirmation of an undeniable form of madness (Becker, 2014; Lélut, 1836). Soon a large number of psychiatrists and other scholars committed to their own studies of geniuses (Galton, 1869; Lange-Eichbaum and Paul, 1931; Lombroso, 1891; Maudsley, 1908), and within a century there was a large literature on genius and in particular genius and madness. Most of the authors of this literature argued for the genius as pathological, a view especially held by the burgeoning psychiatric field, while those challenging the mad genius stand were more often psychologists stressing that physical and emotional stability rather than illness was associated with genius (Becker, 1978).

A shift in interest and the rebirth of biological psychiatry

Becker argues that the considerable interest in the mad genius question waned during the mid-twentieth century in parallel with an opposition to eugenics. Increasingly environmental factors were argued for in the development of the genius. The change from a biological to a sociological stance was manifested in a change of language; studies on genius were now supplanted with studies on creativity, intelligence and motivation (Becker, 1978; Lehman, 1947). While Becker is certainly accurate in the shift of interest from a biological to a sociological standpoint during the first half of the twentieth century, it is not true that studies on genetics and creativity or, for that matter, on creativity and psychiatric disorder decreased. In fact studies on creativity and genetics has seen a steady increase from the beginning of the twentieth century until today (see Chapter 5 of this book for a thorough review), while a similar increase has also been observed within the field of creativity and psychopathology (Thys et al., 2014b). The 1970s and 1980s saw the re-emergence of a biological psychiatry paralleled with a substantial increase in studies of creativity and psychopathology (Karlsson, 1970; Shorter, 1997); however, the number of scientific studies on creativity and psychopathology has consistently doubled each decade from two studies in the 1950s to 41 studies in the first decade of the twenty-first century (Thys et al., 2014b).

Many of these studies have suggested an association for bipolar disorder and creativity (Andreasen, 1987; Jamison, 1989; Kyaga et al., 2013; Kyaga et al., 2011; Ludwig, 1995; Richards et al., 1988). Increasingly there has been a growing consensus that there is an association between creative abilities and mental illness resting on a biological foundation resulting in an inherent disposition. As Becker notes (2014), the modern conception of bipolar spectrum traits has many similarities with ancient ideas of temperament. Nevertheless, it is important to remind oneself of the main argument of this chapter: the idea of the mad genius was born in antiquity, but has changed considerably over history stressing both rationality and unrestricted imagination at its core.

3
Early Empirical Studies of Genius

Introduction

Louis Lélut presented the first medical examination of genius in 1836 (Becker, 2014; Lélut, 1836). There followed a large number of studies on geniuses (Galton, 1869; Lange-Eichbaum and Paul, 1931; Lombroso, 1891; Maudsley, 1908), and soon the literature on genius and in particular genius and madness was comprehensive. The author foremost associated with the idea of the mad genius during this period was the Italian psychiatrist Cesare Lombroso (1835–1909). In *The Man of Genius*, Lombroso argues for genius being inevitably linked to madness and degeneration (Lombroso, 1891). His contemporary, Francis Galton (1822–1911) was not convinced of this view but forcefully argued for traits of genius being hereditary. In what is often suggested the birth of behavioural genetics, *Hereditary Genius: An enquiry into its laws and consequences*, he makes a compelling argument for genius being hereditary by collecting data from renowned English families. The emphasis on factors of genius unsusceptible to alteration was increasingly questioned, however, and in 1928 Wilhelm Lange-Eichbaum (1875–1949) contended a sociological perspective on the definition of genius. In an English shortened version of his immense *Genie – Irrsinn und Ruhm*, he asserts that, 'The one who is not yet called a genius is no genius' (Lange-Eichbaum and Paul, 1931, p. 67). Nevertheless, he says, 'It cannot be a chance matter that among geniuses the healthy constitute a minority' (p. 125). This later assertion was substantiated in a study of artists and scientists by Adele Juda published in 1949. The present chapter investigates some of the early studies, focusing on the studies by Lombroso, Galton, Lange-Eichbaum and Juda.

Cesare Lombroso

Cesare Lombroso was born 6 November, 1835, in Verona, Italy, into a wealthy Jewish family (Carra and Barale, 2004; Knepper and Ystehede, 2013). He studied medicine at the University of Pavia and graduated in 1858 with a thesis on endemic cretinism in Lombardy. Lombroso spent his early career in southern Italy working as a medical officer in an infantry fighting brigandage (robbery and plunder). He successively developed a deep interest in the behavioural characteristics of brigands. Consequently, in 1863 he returned to the University of Pavia and became the first professor of mental disease studies. In 1872 he published *Genio e Follia [The Man of Genius]*, and caused a sensation, arguing that the genius is a degenerate whose insanity is an evolutionary compensation for excessive intellectual progress (1891).

His best-known work, *L'uomo delinquent [The Criminal Man]*, is regarded as the birth of modern criminology (Carra and Barale, 2004; Lombroso, 1911). By reviewing the autopsies of criminals, he held that certain physical stigmata (e.g., a deviation in head size and shape, eye defects, pouches in the cheeks like those of some animals, the abundance, variety, and precocity of wrinkles) were suggestive of a biological predisposition to commit crimes.

Lombroso's ideas on criminality have been discredited by modern science, but his ideas had the importance of stressing *scientific* study of the criminal mind, directing attention on the criminal rather than the crime. He consistently underscored the need for direct study of the individual, using objective measurements and statistical methods, reflecting the basic idea of cause as a chain of interrelated events (Maj and Ferro, 2002).

Lombroso is also interesting in the sense that he represents a part of the *Jewish social science* that emerged in the late nineteenth century in response to increasing anti-Semitism (Knepper and Ystehede, 2013). Proponents of anti-Semitism adhered to this term to emphasize that they were not opposed to Jews for religious reasons, but rather because of their racial characteristics. Anti-Semitic ideas were flourishing in Germany and Austria with political parties contesting for elections, and in France with the Dreyfus affair exposing a latent anti-Semitism. In the United States and the United Kingdom anti-Semitic rhetoric was raised owing to immigrants fleeing Russian pogroms and increasing Jewish communities in urban areas. While many of Lombroso's ideas echo thoughts finally leading to the holocaust, his ideas were in fact commonly held by a group of Jewish social scientists as arguments *against* anti-Semitism. Jewish intellectuals, such as Joseph Jacobs, Arthur Ruppin, and Maurice Fishberg, used the measurements of skulls, noses, and chests to argue the superiority of the *Jewish race* compared to other races. Joseph Jacobs who first attracted public recognition through articles in *The Times* drawing attention to Russian persecution of Jews, later insisted that the remarkable similarity of Jewish physiognomy all over the world implied *racial purity* (Knepper and Ystehede, 2013). He argued that the comparative anthropological evidence pointed to a race with *superior* mental capacity, evidenced by the prevalence of Jews in European dictionaries of eminent individuals. Similar opinions were held by Max Nordau with his highly influential *Degeneration* published in 1892 (1892/1993), and also illustrated in *The Man of Genius* by Lombroso (1891). On the influence of race and heredity for genius and insanity Lombroso writes, 'owing to the bloody selection of mediaeval persecutions, and owing also to the influence of temperate climate, the Jews of Europe have risen above those of Africa and the East, and have often surpassed the Aryans. It is not only a difference in general culture, but we find more precocious and extended mental work applied to different sciences. It is certainly thus in music, the drama, satirical and humorous literature, journalism, and in various branches of science. This has been statistically proven by various writers, as by Jacobs in a very careful study on the ability of the Jews in Western Europe and of Jews in general' (p. 133).

It is therefore important to recognize that Lombroso's and other writings emphasizing genetic and hereditary factors of genius during the turn of the century cannot be dismissed as simple anti-Semitic propaganda, but should rather be seen as a general focus of study, finally leading up to the atrocious consequences of eugenics. For obvious reasons then the hereditary framework in general as well as the mad genius link was considerably downplayed following the Second World War. Still, *The Man of Genius* made a lasting impact on the public's apprehension of genius inevitably linked to madness.

The characteristics of genius

Lombroso begins his book with the usual historical reference to Aristotle, and suggesting that 'even genius, the one human power before which we may bow the knee without shame, has been classed by not a few alienists as on the confines of criminality, one of the teratologic forms of the human mind, a variety of insanity' (p. 2). He then turns to describe some of the main characteristics of geniuses in his opinion, e.g., height, rickets, pallor, cranium, left-handedness, as well as psychological traits.

On height, he claims that most geniuses were of short stature, such as Horace, Alexander the great, Aristotle, Plato, Linneaus, Spinoza, Mozart, Balzac, Ibsen, and many others, whereas only a few were tall: among others Volta, Schiller, and Flaubert. Many were hunch-backed, or club-footed and pallid. Lombroso devotes considerable space for descriptions of the cranium and the brains of geniuses arguing also that many geniuses had lesions of the head and brain. He argues that stammering as well as left-handedness is frequent among geniuses. While most of these ideas seem antiquated today, there is some evidence for an association between left-handedness and creative abilities (Preti and Vellante, 2007).

With regards to psychological traits, Lombroso suggests that geniuses are characterized by a strong apprehension of their own new ideas, but quickly disregard new ideas by others. They are driven by instinct and inspiration, and subjected to an almost 'perverted' sensibility. Many, especially if men of science, 'occupy themselves throughout their whole lives with one single problem' (p. 32), referred to as *monotypic mania*. The sensibility and the monotypic mania renders geniuses 'very difficult to persuade or dissuade ... In them the roots of error, as well as those of truth, fix themselves more deeply and multiplexly than in other men, for whom opinion is a habit, an affair of fashion, or of circumstance. Hence the slight utility of moral treatment as applied to the insane; hence also the frequent fallibility of genius'.

The psychological traits described by Lombroso in geniuses are in the main supported by modern creativity research. In general, the literature supports that creative individuals are characterized by a strong belief in their own ideas (Feist, 1998; Nelson, 2007), paired with a high sensibility (Runco, 2007a). They are more impulsive (Feist, 1998). Successful artists also tend to be persistent (Csikszentmihalyi, 1996), which some argue is necessary for high-level accomplishment regardless of domain (Simon, 1988). However, it does not seem that creative individuals are characterized by a *rigid* focus on a single problem, rather they demonstrate endurance over a long period of time, even a lifetime, with considerable more flexibility and variation in behaviour for specific means and goals (Runco, 2007a). In a study on creative architects compared to less creative colleagues, MacKinnon suggests that, 'the more creative architects, more often than the less creative, point turning to another activity when seriously blocked at a task and returning later to it when refreshed, whereas less creative architects more often report working stubbornly at a problem when blocked in their attempts at solutions' (MacKinnon, 1965 quoted in Runco, 2007a). Nevertheless, the difficulty in persuading creative individuals alluded to by Lombroso may also rest in the fact that many tend to be *contrarians*, a term used for people who do things different from others (Runco, 2007a).

The causes of genius

The second part of Lombroso's book revolves around the causes of genius. These are summarized into meteorology, climate, race and heredity, disease, and civilization. With regards to the weather, Lombroso arrives after describing the chronology of several 'men of geniuses' that the temperature and weather is of significant importance with regards to accomplishments in both artistic and scientific areas. He suggests that artistic and literary creations reach their maximum in the spring, while great physical, chemical and mathematical discoveries are also mostly made in the spring. Out of 1871 discoveries investigated by Lombroso, 541 were made in spring, 485 in autumn, 477 in the summer, 368 in winter. He commented 'It is evident, then, that the first warm months distinctly predominate in the creations of genius ... in the spring that the discovery of America was conceived, as well as galvanism, the barometer, the telescope, and the lightning conductor; in the spring, Michelangelo had the idea of his great cartoon, Dante of his *Divina Commedia*, Leonardo of his book on light, Goethe of his *Faust'* (p. 113). Lombroso links this increase of accomplishments during spring to his own studies of patients committed to asylum in Italy and a similar French study by Esquirol, arguing for a parallel increase of patients entering asylums with the increase of accomplishments.

It is of course easy to dismiss Lombroso's findings on the grounds of his probable biased selection of accomplishments. However, there is now evidence for seasonality in mood disorders, and more specifically bipolar disorder. A recent large-scale study conducted in Taiwan demonstrated a significant spring/summer increase of admissions to psychiatric care for mania, which has previously been demonstrated in smaller studies (Lee et al., 2007; Symonds and Williams, 1976). There is also some evidence that prominent writers are more susceptible to seasonal sensitivity than are the general population, although this was not linked to increased creativity (Barbato et al., 2007).

Lombroso continues to argue that aspects such as warm climate and lower air pressure in hilly areas is important for the development of geniuses; arguments, such as the presence of anaerobic microbes and ozonized air to influence the brain of geniuses. All these seem questionable at least.

Next come aspects of race and heredity in the formation of geniuses. As previously described, Lombroso contends that the 'Jewish race' is exceptional in producing a high frequency of geniuses. But, he also argues that they display a high grade of insanity. Referring to studies by Jacobs, Lombroso claims that it is 'curious to note that the Jewish elements in the population furnish four and even six times as many lunatics as the rest of the population' (p. 136), thus linking genius with insanity. However, this is not true of Jews alone, claims Lombroso, who also quotes Beard commenting that 'the neurotic tendency which dominates North America makes of that country a land of great orators' (p. 137).

The hereditary aspects of genius is addressed by describing pedigrees of some historical geniuses and by referring to the work of Galton (see this chapter), of which Lombroso says, 'Galton, in a work of great value, but in which he often commits the mistake (from which I cannot free myself) of confusing talent with genius' (p. 141). This differentiation is further stressed by Wilhelm Lange-Eichbaum in his study of sociological aspects of genius (see this chapter), and still prevails today in creativity research (see Chapter 4 on big-C and little-c) (Lange-Eichbaum, 1928; Lange-Eichbaum and Paul, 1931; Runco, 2007a).

Lombroso still suggests that the hereditary aspects of genius put forward by Galton are bleak in comparison to the hereditary aspects of 'insanity'. This may also be said to hold today. Modern estimates of heritability in creativity range from 22 per cent (Nichols, 1978) to 78 per cent (Barron, 1970), while most estimates of heritability in severe psychiatric disorders are around 60–80 per cent (Sadock et al., 2009). Chapter 5 more thoroughly discusses heritability estimates of creativity.

The question of somatic disease in genius is discussed briefly by Lombroso. He quotes Maine de Biran saying that, 'when a man does not suffer he does not think of himself; disease alone and the habit of reflection enable us to distinguish ourselves' (p. 151). This idea, that somatic disease facilitates genius is not supported in more contemporary investigations. Post, in his study of 291 world-famous men, argues that when having 'survived the hazards of late 18th century and 19th century childhoods, these outstanding men would seem to have been much healthier than most of their contemporaries: 41% enjoyed robust health, and only 8% had been plagued by debilitating illnesses' (1994).

Turning to social influences, Lombroso tends to downplay these in favour of hereditary factors and climate. While he acknowledges that 'Greece, placed in ancient times by race and nature in the first rank, as regards to intellectual creation, no longer shows any trace of her superiority. Nature and the race have not changed, but slavery, political struggles, and hard living have exhausted all her strength', still holds that 'It appears to me that, in many cases, social influences are more apparent than real – analogous rather to the peck of the chicken which cracks the egg-shell than to the spermatozoid which generates the embryo' (pp. 154–5). In essence, Lombroso feels that social factors such as urbanization and opportunity are 'only the last drop which make the vessel run over. This is so true that the cases in which genius has manifested itself in spite of adverse circumstances and even violent opposition, are innumerable'.

As we shall see, this view was already being questioned in the beginning of the twentieth century by Lange-Eichbaum (Lange-Eichbaum and Paul, 1931), and this discussion has continued today (Sawyer, 2010). The relative impact of nature and nurture in the formation of genius has been extensively discussed by the well-known psychologist, Hans Eysenck in addressing the problem of *causal* elements in relation to risk factors for the formation of genius as well as for complex phenomena in general (1995). Causes must be both necessary and sufficient, while risk factors are only correlated, and not necessarily causally related, to the variable investigated. While, for example, there is agreement that both in historical and present time most creative individuals, regardless of discipline, have come from middle or upper-middle classes, this is a correlation not necessarily causally related to genius.

Genius in the insane

The third part of *The Man of Genius*, embarks on a historical journey of 'insane genius' in literature and art. On poets, Lombroso writes, 'Their most salient characteristic – originality heightened to the point of absurdity – is due to overflowing of the imagination which can no longer be restrained within the bounds of logic and common sense' (p. 171). For artists, Lombroso refers to work done by others, in which together with his own, a '108 mental patients with artistic tendencies, of which: – 46 were towards painting, 10 sculpture, 11 engraving, 8 music, 5 architecture, 28 poetry' were investigated (p. 179). Based on findings in this group, Lombroso argues that only few had their mental tendencies due to the professions, but rather that the mental inclination came first. The works of these artists were generally characterized by, e.g., symbolism, minuteness of detail and absurdity. He then goes on to characterize the choice of subject specifically influenced by the type of malady suffered. For example, he suggests that, 'Alcoholic maniacs often make an excessive use of yellow in their pictures' (p. 181). Insane artists are also characterized by their originality, according to Lombroso, but nevertheless 'even originality ends by degenerating, in all, or nearly all, into mere eccentricity, which only seems logical when one enters into the idea of the delusion' (p. 186).

Lombroso also identifies a group of individuals with less severe mental disorders, which he describes as the 'mattoids'. These individuals are quite often offspring to geniuses. He has little positive to say about this group. They seem to lack both competence and insight. 'All topics are welcome to mattoids, even those most foreign to their profession or occupation; but they are found to choose by preference the most grotesque and uncertain subjects, or questions which it is impossible to solve' (p. 220). Yet they 'show a deficiency rather than an exuberance of inspiration; they fill entire volumes, without sense or savour; they eke out the commonplaceness of their ideas and their poverty of style' (p. 214). True genius, according to Lombroso, is found in those with the most severe and 'least curable forms (monomania and moral insanity), together with dementia, and those forms which it accompanies, or in which it is latent (megalomania and paralysis)' (p. 180).

In all, Lombroso's description of literary and artistic genius in relation to mental illness is difficult to characterize as anything other than mere opinions, although to some extent based on empirical material. While this is true, present literature seem to support, in line with Lombroso's suggestions, that heightened creativity is not associated with all forms of psychopathology but rather with the more severe forms (Kyaga et al., 2013). Lombroso's description of mattoids also echoes contemporary criticism of *impressions management*. While it is true that famous creators sometimes aim for self-promotion (Gardner, 1993), Rubenson and Runco suggest that there are much better ways to invest one's time than in impression management if one is interested in cultivating a creative career (1992, 1995).

Synthesis

The final part of Lombroso's book attempts a synthesis of his observations. Some of the main aspects of insane geniuses are summarized into characterlessness, vanity, precocity, alcoholism, vagabondage, versatility, originality, style, religious doubts, sexual abnormities, egoism, eccentricity, and inspiration.

Regarding their lack of character, Lombroso says, 'These insane geniuses have scarcely any character. The full complete character "which bends not for any winds," is the distinctive mark of honest and sound-minded men' (p. 314). While this statement is clearly a blunt oversimplification, the impression may again be explained partly by the fact that many creative individuals tend to be *contrarians* (Runco, 2007a). Similarly, originality and eccentricity may fall into this tendency. Gamman and Raein have recently also suggested some shared traits in creative individuals and criminals, such as in the identification of being an 'outsider' facilitating the opportunity of 'breaking the paradigm' (2010). Lombroso stresses this character of the man of genius 'being essentially original and a lover of originality, is a natural enemy of traditions and conservatism: he is the born revolutionary, the precursor and the most active pioneer of revolutions' (p. 335).

There is some support in the literature for eccentricity and self-promotion (Gardner, 1993), alcoholism (Ludwig, 1992, 1995; Post, 1994, 1996), and fairly good support for precocity and achievement in men of genius (Simonton, 1988a). A general increase in alcohol abuse in artists has been suggested by Ludwig in a study of 1005 outstanding individuals who had their biographies published in the *New York Times* book review from 1960 to 1990 (1992, 1995). Then again, when Ludwig examined writers specifically, alcohol use proved unfavourable to productivity in over 75 per cent of the writers (1990). In general, alcohol abuse in the long run does not seem to be beneficial for creativity (Kyaga, 2014).

More importantly, Lombroso argues that the 'insane characters of men of genius are scarcely ever found alone', but rather that men of genius, like Chopin, Comte and Schopenhauer, demonstrate alternating insanity of melancholia, and 'exaggerated self-esteem' (p. 327). Lombroso summarizes, 'the temper of these men is so different from that of average people that it gives a special character to the different psychoses (melancholia, monomania, etc.) from which they suffer, so as to constitute a special psychosis, which might be called the psychosis of genius' (p. 329). This comment is clearly in line with the bulk of contemporary studies on creativity and mental illness. Most studies affirm an association between bipolar disorder and creative achievements (Thys et al., 2014b).

The final two chapters in Lombroso's book are devoted to the 'epileptoid nature of genius' and 'sane men of genius'. In the first of these chapters, Lombroso refers to confessions of several 'eminent men of genius', such as Buffon and Dostoyevsky. Citing the latter, 'There are moments ... and it is only a matter of five or six seconds – when you suddenly feel the presence of the eternal harmony' (p. 339). The resemblance of inspiration and epilepsy has been suggested by several writers, although there is actually very little empirical support for any association between creativity and epilepsy. Some contemporary studies have addressed different forms of dementia (see Chapter 6), but in all these do not support any sustained increase in creativity (De Souza et al., 2010; Drago et al., 2006; Miller et al., 1998).

For the few geniuses that seem sane, Lombroso settles that in many cases insanity goes unrecognized, and thus these may very well have suffered both insanity and epilepsy, 'who, but for the revelations of some of his intimate friends, would have suspected that Cavour was repeatedly subject to attacks of suicidal mania, or thought that Richelieu was epileptic' (p. 354). Lombroso concludes his book by saying, 'In short, by these analogies, and coincidences between the phenomena of genius and mental aberration, it seems as though nature had intended to teach us respect for the supreme misfortunes of insanity' (p. 361).

Francis Galton

Sir Francis Galton was born the youngest of a family of nine children. His mother, Violetta Darwin, was aunt to Charles Darwin, and Galton's grandfather, Samuel Galton, was a Fellow of the Royal Society (Smith, 1997). Galton's father, Samuel Tertius Galton, directed a bank, and thus the family was a family of means. This was important as young Galton attempted, but failed, both medical school and in his efforts to complete an honours degree in mathematics at Cambridge. However, from an early age he demonstrated great aptitude. In an often quoted letter to his sister Adèle, Galton writes (Forrest, 1974):

> *My dear Adèle,*
> *I am four years old and can read any English book. I can say all the Latin substantives and adjectives and active words besides 52 lines of Latin poetry. I can cast up any sum in addition and multiply by*
> *2, 3, 4, 5, 6, 7, 8, (9), 10, (11)*
> *I can also say the pence table, I read French a little and I know the clock.*
> *Francis Galton*

While lacking in formal mathematics, Galton had an exceptional skill in understanding the meaning of data. He was a brilliant natural statistician (Senn, 2011), with a near obsessive tendency to measure and count the things he experienced in his life. Today we may laugh at his attempts to quantify such immeasurable things as attraction, love, beauty, or the effectiveness of prayer, but in fact Galton essentially founded not one but three or even four entire branches of science – *statistics, psychometrics* (measuring mental faculties), differential psychology, *meteorology* and eugenics, the latter now largely discredited, but reincarnated without its gruesome social implications in *behavioural genetics* (Champkin, 2011). His first published work, however, came comparably late at the age of 28 (Smith, 1997), with his first interests centered on exploration of South West Africa and Egypt, geography, and meteorology. These were subjects that would remain major interests for Galton throughout his life (Smith, 1997). But, it was with his attempt to quantify achievement that he embarked on the first scientific investigation of genius (Galton, 1869). Inspired by both Adolphe Quetelet's *Letters on the Theory of Probabilities* and Charles Darwin's *On the Origin of Species*, Galton assumed that aptitude, just as height and weight, was normally distributed, and hereditary (Darwin, 1859; Quetelet and Beamish, 1839). His research led to the publication of *Hereditary Talent and Character*, two articles in *Macmillan's Magazine* (Galton). This was followed four years later by the book-length treatment of the same subject, *Hereditary Genius: An Inquiry into its laws and consequences* (1869), the aim of which was 'to show ... that a man's natural abilities are derived by inheritance, under exactly the same limitations as are the form and physical features of the whole organic world' (p. 1).

Galton's first problem was how to assess genius. He chose to consider eminence in an occupation as a proxy for mental ability. Claiming that, 'I feel convinced that no man can achieve a very high reputation without being gifted with very high abilities' (p. 49). He then argued that the distribution of mental ability is similarly distributed as physical traits are, such as height and weight. By initially investigating 200 men with mathematical honours at Cambridge Galton concludes (Table 3.1), 'the range of mental power between ... the greatest and least of English intellects is enormous. There is a continuity of natural ability reaching from one knows not what height, and descending to one can hardly say what depth' (p. 26). This continuity made it possible for Galton to estimate the proportion of men anticipated at each level of mental ability ranging from the highest to the lowest, which in turn, provided a baseline for which the heritability of mental ability could be appraised.

Galton then went on to investigate the family backgrounds of those at the highest levels of achievement and consider if these achievements appeared to run within families. He consecutively presented data for judges, statesmen, commanders, literary men, scientists, poets, musicians, painters, divines and others, measuring the occurrences with which eminence among these were found among first (fathers, brothers, sons), second (grandfathers, grandsons, uncles, nephews), and third degree relatives (great-grandfathers, great-grandsons, great-uncles, great-nephews, first cousins). By comparing these numbers with estimates from the general population, he concluded that relatives of eminent men 1) more often were eminent than expected and 2) that the frequency of eminence declined from first to second to third degree relatives. Thus, he came to the conclusion that these findings could only be explained by mental ability being familial.

At the time this was a rather provocative statement, but Galton claimed that his conclusion was supported by data and statistical analysis. In this regard his work was truly pioneering. As Galton himself pronounced, 'The theory of hereditary genius, though usually scouted, has been advocated by a few writers in past as well as in modern times. But I may claim to be the first to treat the subject in a statistical manner, to arrive at numerical results, and to introduce the "law of deviation from an average" into discussions of heredity' (p. iv).

Interestingly, while Galton chose not to approach the idea of genius and madness in *Hereditary Genius*, he later in life suggested this association. In Galton's first biography written by his scientific heir and friend Karl Pearson, Galton claimed, 'there is the fact that men who leave their mark on the world are very often those who, being gifted and full of nervous power, are at the same time haunted and driven by a dominant idea, and are therefore within a measurable distance of insanity. This weakness

Table 3.1 Scale of merit among the men who obtain mathematical honours at Cambridge

Number of marks obtained by candidates	Number of candidates in the two years, taken together, who obtained those marks
Under 500	24
500 to 1,000	74
1,000 to 1,500	38
1,500 to 2,000	21
2,000 to 2,500	11
2,500 to 3,000	8
3,000 to 3,500	11
3,500 to 4,000	5
4,000 to 4,500	2
4,500 to 5,000	1
5,000 to 5,500	3
5,500 to 6,000	1
6,000 to 6,500	0
6,500 to 7,000	0
7,000 to 7,500	0
7,500 to 8,000	1
	200

Source: Adapted from Galton, F., 1869.
Note: The reults of two years are thrown into a single table. The total number of marks obtainable in each year was 17,000.

will probably betray itself occasionally in disadvantageous forms among their descendants. Some of these will be eccentric, others feeble-minded, others nervous, and some may be downright lunatics.' (Pearson, 1914, vol III, p. 32).

Wilhelm Lange-Eichbaum

Wilhelm Lange-Eichbaum was originally a sculptor and an author of plays, but later devoted his life to the study of psychiatry as a student of Gaupp's renowned school at the University of Tuebingen (Loewenberg, 1950; Mayer, 1953). He worked at the University of Hamburg, where he aimed to establish pathography as a science, investigating both biological and sociological influences on disease. His vast *Genie – Irrsin und Ruhm* published in 1928, including biographies of 800 geniuses, challenged many of those ideas presented in Lombroso's and Galton's works. *The Problem of Genius*, an English condensation of *Genie – Irrsin und Ruhm*, highlighting Lange-Eichbaum's ideas on the mad genius question was published in 1931. In a preface by Paul Cedar, Lange-Eichbaum is said to maintain that 'Talent is the hereditary endowment which will enable an individual, should circumstances became favourable, to fulfil particular tasks (mathematical, musical, sculptural, etc.)'; however, *genius* is not 'a mysterious form of hereditary equipment provided once for all at birth' (p. x). Rather the 'individual is only the bearer, the sustainer of genius. He (or she) is usually talented but not necessarily so, and becomes famous through a fortunate concatenation of circumstances' (p. x). Lange-Eichbaum claims that 'In a word, a genius is one who is revered by numerous persons. There is no such thing as a distinct human type which can be labelled genius, for genius is only a social relationship, the relationship of the bearer of genius to mankind ... One who is not yet called a genius is not a genius' (p. x).

Lange-Eichbaum himself clearly states that he attempts to address the question of genius by using an empirical approach:

> What does every investigator do when confronted by whatever problem you like to think of? He tranquilly contemplates reality; he allows things, as they appear, to influence him; and then he does his best to depict and to describe the phenomenal world. Only when this has been accomplished does he begin to search in the multiplicity for the common elements, the ruling principles, the 'laws'. Then, as a third step, he will proceed to fit these principles and laws into the framework of his general outlook on the universe, of his philosophy.

Such is the method adopted to-day by every physicist, chemist, biologist, and psychologist.

What has hitherto been the universal way of studying genius? Hundreds upon hundreds of investigators have adopted the very opposite method. Setting out from their philosophy, from their general outlook upon the universe, they sought a solution for the problem of genius with the aid of their meta-physics. They constructed out of their own ideals regulating the appearance of genius. Living reality was indifferent to them; what could not be fitted into the framework of their theory was not 'true' genius. That is why nearly all extant theories of genius contradict one another. Each investigator describes it in accordance with his own ideals. (p. 3).

These words, today still have bearing on the discussion of the mad genius link. Contemporary authors tend to take contradictory positions holding everything from mental illness having nothing to do with creativity to others arguing for it being intimately linked: opinions that rarely are based on empirical studies (Silvia and Kaufman, 2010).

Lange-Eichbaum provides the necessary historical framework for the definition of genius, telling that the glorification of the genius as someone exhibiting creative energy first took hold in the Italian Renaissance. However, 'To make the genius an ideal of personality is characteristic of the bourgeois epoch. In paying homage to the productive writer and the sculptor, the bourgeois is, as it were, paying homage to himself, is elevating his own nobility, intellectual nobility, to the rank of an ideal' (p. 6). Focusing on the relativity of genius, Lange-Eichbaum suggests that the difficulties in acknowledging who is truly a genius mean that, 'a hundred different persons will compile a hundred different lists, giving pride of place, now to Plato, now to Dante, now to Colombus or to Shakespeare, now to Goethe ... No two lists will be identical' (p. 8). Therefore there is the need of, 'an abstract formula which will lift us above the plane of all these contradictions, while remaining valid for each particular instance. That is the crucial problem of genius' (p. 11). He argues that it is clear that genius must be the result of valuation, that, in lack of absolute values, genius must be reflected in the relation between the genius – the object – and the subject valuing it. This value emanates from an *enjoyment factor*, with admirers being the consumers of this factor; thus 'A genius is a bringer of spiritual values, and one who is revered by numerous persons' (p. 14).

Lange-Eichbaum separates the genius, and the achievements made. He exemplifies with the many inventors that go unrecognized though their inventions have changed the lives of many. The reason for this is that the value of the invention is *objective*; the personality of its creator is therefore indifferent to us, while the work of artists and founders of religion instead are more esteemed. This is because such work is subjective and inherently related to its creator. The potential genius must also exhibit certain features 'to impress or influence the masses of mankind' (p. 18). These are, first, an impression of *superiority*, which is usually aroused by exceptional talent. Second, the admirer needs to be moved by a sense of forceful, almost compulsive, *passion*, echoing Galton's suggestion of exceptional drive. Third, is *charm* and allurement, because 'as we admire, we enjoy a flattering elevation of our own ego'. Fourth, and most importantly, the admirer wants to be *astonished*, wants to see miracles, something characterizing works of great art. Juxtaposed to these four aspects, is a fifth *negative* one: 'The sinister or uncanny may manifest itself in the work, in the character traits, and above all in the life-history of the genius. Suffering may be his reward. Our horror of the unmeaning makes his value shine all the more brightly before our eyes. Though it be unconsciously, we love most of all to see a genius wearing the martyr's crown', providing a clue to the historical notion of genius and madness.

While Lange-Eichbaum suggests that hereditary endowment may be an important factor in propelling an individual into fame, and finally general acclaim of being a genius, he also clearly states that talent is not a necessary prerequisite: 'we shall find that all possible human types can be raised to the rank of genius, all conceivable varieties and grades of talent, of half-talent, or of no talent at all. We shall find persons who psychologically and biologically are thoroughly different one from another. There are thousand kinds of inborn talent, but there is no such thing as a distinct human type which can be labelled genius' (p. 25).

Necessary is, according to Lange-Eichbaum, for the burgeoning genius to acquire *fame*, 'a reputation for genius must be preceded by positive fame' (p. 33). However, 'Only in rare instances does fame lead to the appraisement of the famous person as a genius ... It is a rare variety of fame, a climax of fame, thanks to which the individual is felt, with a certain ardour, to have something sacred about him, and is thus enshrined as a "genius"'. It follows then that, 'One who is not yet called a genius is not a genius. "Unrecognised" genius does not exist; people are not geniuses until they have been "recognized"'. This recognition is made by both 'leading authorities, but partly by simple folk, by the broad masses' (p. 67). And it may also fluctuate over time, something Lange-Eichbaum argues does not implicate that, 'The "judgement of posteriority" is "more just" or "more accurate" than that of contemporaries; it is merely different', a reflection which 'brings us face to face with the problem of creative talent' (p. 68).

Lange-Eichbaum goes to some length to discern genius from talent: 'Talent is the hereditary endowment which will enable an individual, should circumstances become favourable, to fulfil particular tasks (mathematical, musical, sculptural, etc.). Strictly speaking, therefore, it is only a "potential" endowment, but such endowments are part of the inborn psycho-biological constitution. They do not, however, in themselves constitute a capacity for achievement' (p. 72). 'Talent of this order is always something organic, biological, constitutional, for it is very markedly hereditary. We must, however, guard against looking upon this hereditary equipment as localised in concrete masses of the brain.' (p. 73). 'The person thus endowed will be more likely than the other to become a genius.' (p. 74). 'When there is very high endowment for creative achievement, we regard the talent as exceptional. The history of certain families with marked musical or mathematical gifts proves beyond question that such exceptional talents are hereditary' (p. 75). Lange-Eichbaum also suggests that the 'biological type of creative worker gives to his work as a whole its character, its tint, and its trend' (p. 78), with a division between the 'dreamy and romantic person ... and abstract systematisers; predominantly rationalist in their outlook'. This idea has consistently resurfaced through the study of the mad genius link, and there is also some empirical support for this division with regards to psychopathology (Campbell and Wang, 2012; Jamison, 2000; Kyaga et al., 2013; Sass, 2000a, 2000b).

The fourth chapter of *The Problem of Genius* is entirely devoted to the question of *genius and insanity*. Here Lange-Eichbaum contends: '"Genius and insanity" – the dispute which has raged over this theme reminds us of a sphinx with a Medusa's head. For two and a half thousand years attempts have been made to answer the riddle. They have been futile. As long as people continued to regard geniuses as a biologically recognisable variety of human beings, as long as they clung to the arbitrary theories of particular thinkers, as long as they failed to recognise that geniuses are created by mankind at large and that the making of a genius is a sociological process of becoming – just so long it was inevitable that those who tried to study genius should grope in the dark. But as soon as we agree to contemplate genius sociologically, light flashes on the ancient problem' (p. 102).

Thus, he holds that his approach may solve the ancient question by at the very least acknowledging the difference between *talent* and *genius*.

Referring to Lombroso, he says, 'The implication of the title of the book [Lombroso's *The Man of Genius*] is that every genius is in some way insane or degenerate. Is this so? Are there really no sane or healthy geniuses? Actual experience shows that this may happen ... There is not an invariable or necessary association of genius with insanity. None the less, the detailed psychiatric investigations of the last hundred years show with irrefutable cogency that among geniuses healthy persons form a small minority' (p. 110). Lange-Eichbaum then turns to quantitative data to support this argument on the basis of the pathographies he has performed:

> When we study the entire population of the country [Germany] with reference to the existence of mental disorders, we find that from 0.2 to 0.3 per cent are under restraint in asylums, and that a fairly high estimate, not more than about 0.5 per cent of the total population will be affected with grave mental disorder.
>
> But among geniuses (considered to the number of three to four hundred individuals) we find that from 12 to 13 per cent have been psychotic at least once during their lifetime. Confining our examinations to the 'very greatest' names, numbering seventy-eight in all, we find that more than 37 per cent have been psychotic once during their lifetime; that more than 83 per cent have been markedly psychopathic. (p. 112).

Acknowledging that the question of an association between *genius* and *insanity* is complicated, Lange-Eichbaum says 'It cannot be a chance matter that among geniuses the healthy constitute a minority' (p. 125), and contends that five statements can be made with reasonable assurance: 1) most geniuses have never been psychotic (severe psychiatric disorder), but psychopathic (less severe psychiatric disorder), 2) many of those suffering psychopathy have suffered nervous tensions, 3) have been given to drink and drug-habits, and 4) have manifested certain exceptional mental states, e.g., a craze for creation or ecstasy, 5) and in cases where there has been genuine psychosis, a causal connection to creative activity has seldom been found (p. 116).

The reason for most geniuses having been psychopaths, says Lange-Eichbaum, is because 'the psychopathic taint has transformed them in a peculiar way that they seem so new, so striking, and bring possibilities of original experience to hundreds of thousands of persons ... because of the primitive and dreamlike character of its thought, the psycho-pathological seems more obscure, and therefore more profound – qualities which have always proved more effective and more lastingly famous than healthy clarity' (p. 131). The psychopathic trait may then further augment the genius in two ways. The first is that it may evolve into a more severe psychosis, thus setting upon the individual's 'head the thorny crown of a victim for the sake of humanity' (p. 132), or the psychopathic qualities of the individual may result in his coming into conflict with society. The latter may then result in later times recognizing him as having 'unparalleled boldness, a manifestation of the spirit of the unconquerable titan' (p. 133). In either case, a *martyr* or a *titan*, he captures the fame necessary for being declared a genius.

Lange-Eichbaum claims statistical evidence for the pathological causation more often providing progress from the 'preliminary stage of celebrity' to the fame of genius, 'The strange and uncanny, the fundamentally unusual, the horror-provoking elements which are hidden away in the morbid personality and work themselves out in the destiny of the individual thus affected, arouse in the observer an impression of something mirum-tremendum, genuinely metaphysical, daimonic, and superhuman' (p. 139). He concludes, that between the three ladders leading to genius; between the *individual* and *achievement*, between *achievement* and *fame*, and finally between *fame* and *genius* there is evidence of morbid factors having causal efficacy, 'Need we be surprised that the upshot of our investigation is that genius is much more often associated with "insanity" than with mental health?'.

Lange-Eichbaum's work can be seen as a substantial advance on the ideas presented by Lombroso and Galton. He adds several layers to the simplified description of the man of genius, as an inborn mental trait. While acknowledging that talent is hereditary, aligning with Galton, he rejects Lombroso's sweeping ideas of genius as degenerate by necessity. He provides a sociological perspective on the evolvement of genius, and forebodes future studies by dissecting talent from genius, while building his ideas on empirics. However, as will be further discussed, unfortunately, Lange-Eichbaum does not provide a clear description on the selection of geniuses that he bases his research on. We are simply told that these are 'über 800 Einzel-Bio-Graphien' (1928), and given a list of some 160 'berühmtheiten'. Despite this weakness, Lange-Eichbaum succeeds in painting a much more nuanced picture of the association between genius and madness; not every genius is insane, but more seem to be than would be expected.

Adele Juda

Lombroso's suggestion of genius inexorably linked to madness had been questioned also before Lange-Eichbaum by, for example, Havelock Ellis in his study of 1030 British geniuses, where he argued for *gout* being surprisingly frequent but with regards to 'insanity' held (Ellis, 1904):

we find that the ascertainable number of cases of insanity is 44, so that the incidence of insanity among our 1 030 eminent persons is 4.2 per cent.

It is perhaps a high proportion. I do not know the number of cases among persons of the educated classes living to a high average age in which it can be said that insanity has occurred at least once during life ... The association of genius with insanity is not, I believe, without significance, but in face of the fact that its occurrence is only demonstrable in less than 5 per cent cases, we must put out of court any theory as to genius being a form of insanity. (p. 191)

However, a final blow to Lombroso's ideas was provided in 1949 by Adele Juda in her study of 294 highly gifted artists and scientists, springing from an investigation of ~19000 individuals of German descent between 1650 and 1900. About 5000 individuals were interviewed. There were 113 artists and 181 scientists. The geographic boundaries were those of Germany prior to the First World War; German Austria, German Switzerland, and the Baltic States. The aim was among others to perform 'a comparison between the mental health of artists and scientists and an average population of similar professional, educational, and social make-up'. Artists consisted of architects, sculptors, poets, painters and musicians, while that scientific group included those active within theoretical science, natural science, technical applied science, and nine statesmen. Results demonstrated that 2.7 per cent of the artists suffered schizophrenia, while this was present among 0.85 per cent in the general population. There was a total absence of 'manic-depressive psychosis' in the artistic group. The main finding was that of the 113 artists, 72 were 'psychically normal', refuting Lombroso's claim of insanity inevitably linked to genius (Lombroso, 1891).

With regards to the high incidence of less severe psychopathology affecting in total a third of artists, Juda suggested that 'The very genesis of the complicated psychic pattern of artists *favours* the concomitant formation of gene combinations which result in a psychopathic disposition. It may be argued that certain qualities such as hypersensitivity, rapidly changing emotions, and even depressive inner experiences had, in some instances, a stimulating effect on the activation of creative ideas'. Brothers and sisters to artists more often exhibited psychopathology than the general population: 'The number of schizophrenics corresponds to the general population, whereas the manic-depressives are twice as frequent as in the average population and the total figure for endogenous insanity is definitely higher than in average people. The low figure for imbeciles, on the other hand, is remarkable'. With regards to children of artists, 'The incidence of endogenous psychoses was 4.1% and definitely increased as compared with 2% of the average population'. Further investigating the 246 adult offspring of artists demonstrated that 21.5% had a cyclothymic constitution and 13.4% schizothymic constitution, suggesting 'a predominance of the cyclothymic temper in the families of the highly gifted artists'.

Among scientists, findings were reversed to those in artists, with an absence of schizophrenia and 3.9 per cent (7 individuals of 181) suffering 'manic-depressive insanity' compared to 0.4 per cent in the average population. Juda comments, 'In manic-depressive psychosis ... we find suppression of creative activity during the attack but revival of the original intellectual power during intermission ... This raises the question of a certain correlation between the cyclothymic constitution and the highest mental ability'. With regards to siblings and children of scientists, they exhibited similar rates of psychopathology as did the relatives of artists.

Finally, Juda investigated 115 artists and scientists of 'higher above-average intellect' but not considered geniuses, during the era of the Second World War. The aim was to capture an intermediate group. Results demonstrated that this group suffered schizophrenia (1.3 per cent) and 'manic-depressive psychosis' (1.3 per cent) less frequently than the highly gifted group, but more frequently than the average population.

Juda summarized her findings in 12 points: 1) there is no definite relationship between highest mental capacity and psychic illness, 2) the geniuses were not at a disadvantage compared to the general population with regards to life duration, fertility, organic diseases, 3) there seems to be a tendency for high mental faculty to manifest itself in first- and second-born children, 4) the families of geniuses do not die out, reflected by the 'remarkable high' number of intellectually prominent children and grandchildren of geniuses, 5) the process by nature of making a genius is complex, but 'direct hereditary transmission is probable in the fields of music, painting, mathematics, and technical invention', 6) eminent artistic talents often displayed capability in combinations of artistic expression, such as music and poetry, 7) the schizothymic constitution is more prevalent among artists, whereas the cyclothymic constitution is more common among scientists, especially among those in the natural sciences, 8) 'the geniuses and their families show a much higher incidence of psychosis and psychoneurosis than the average population. Among the geniuses themselves, schizophrenia occurred only in the artists, and manic-depressive insanity only in the scientists, in a frequency 10 times the incidence of the average population', 9) comparing artists with scientists revealed that artists suffered more 'psychic abnormalities' and more often were single, 10) the 'incidence of below-average intellect and imbecility is remarkably low in descendants of geniuses, whereas the suicide rate appears high', 11) wives to male geniuses contributed directly or indirectly to the accomplishments of their husbands, and 12) the greatest total number of geniuses within German-speaking boundaries 'came from thickly populated and racially mixed middle regions of Germany and Switzerland'.

4
The Development of Modern Creativity Research

Introduction

While many excellent studies on creativity had been published before 1950, modern creativity research has much to credit Joy Paul (J.P.) Guilford, who made creativity a vital subject for researchers in psychology (Runco, 2004). Speaking as their new president at the American Psychological Association (1950), Guilford proposed that creativity was essential for human society. He argued that research in creativity harboured possibilities of great benefit for society. The title of his speech was 'Creativity', and with it, as well as with his subsequent empirical efforts, Guilford managed to convince and persuade researchers that creativity could be approached scientifically (Runco, 2004). His determination sparked the rise of modern creativity research. Many prominent researchers have since attempted to approach the question. As the late Hans Eysenck put it, 'From the beginning of my becoming acquainted with the literature on intelligence, I had been convinced that it was possible to study this concept scientifically. Critics tended to point out that there were important aspects of cognition that seemed to be beyond the scope of science, and creativity and genius were among those most frequently mentioned. Having many other research areas to interest me and take up time and energy, I tried not to think about these topics, but finally temptation became too strong, and I succumbed ... and started to theorize about creativity, and by extension genius' (1995).

Guilford also endorsed the use of psychometrics, the measurement of creativity objectively, and maintained that *divergent thinking* was at the centre of the creative process. Divergent thinking reflects the capability to come up with a wide array of possible solutions to an open-ended problem (Runco, 2010). While Guilford's stress of divergent thinking as a central aspect of creativity has been disputed in recent research, his influence is still evident in the field. Prominent creativity scholars of today have continued Guilford's argument for divergent thinking as a fundamental aspect of creativity (Runco, 2010), not least since the application of divergent thinking has the benefit of being practical compared to other approaches. Other researchers have emphasized other aspects of creativity. For example, a fundamental difference has been made between genius and everyday creativity, also referred to as big-C and little-c, respectively (Kozbelt et al., 2010). While this division was the consequence of lengthy debates in the eighteenth century, they are often used interchangeably in everyday language. However, from a research perspective these two aspects are often investigated with completely different methods. Research in big-C is often centred on creative products, whereas research in little-c often is directed on the subjective experience of the creative process (Kozbelt et al., 2010). The latter is not least considering the frequent lack of products emanating from everyday creativity. In comparison, the judgement of genius is often the consequence of eminent products, such as literature, art or inventions.

The creative *process* and *product* are together with *personality* and *press*, often referred to as the four Ps of creativity research (Kozbelt et al., 2010). Research on personality attempts to identify traits revealing or being contraindicative for creative behaviours. For example, creative artists and scientists share aspects of personality reflected in greater openness to new experiences, ambition and reduced conventionality, and conscientiousness, compared to both less creative colleagues and the average population (Feist, 1998). Hypotheses based on the creative process are often segregated into different stages. Of these, one of the most widespread is by Wallas from 1926 separating the creative process into the four stages: *preparation, incubation, illumination* and *verification*. Research aimed at creative products has the benefit of more straightforwardly allowing a quantitative approach counting, for example, the number of publications, inventions, etc. Therefore creative products are frequently assessed in psychometric studies. Finally, creativity is contingent on the setting, which is addressed in studies of press (from pressures). For instance, creativity usually grows in a milieu providing both resources and tolerance (Florida, 2002).

Genius and everyday creativity

In approaching research on creativity, and specifically research addressed at its association to psychopathology, it is important to note the major difference in conducting research on genius (big-C) compared to much more modest creative achievements (little-c) (Kozbelt et al., 2010). While the unequivocal greatness of works of known artists and scientists is intuitively regarded as creative achievements (big-C), we all in our lives depend on a certain amount of creativity.

This everyday creativity (little-c) has been described by Ruth Richards as 'throughout our lives; it is fundamental to our survival. It is how we find a lost child, get enough to eat, and make our way in a new place and culture. It is not so much what we do as how we do it, whether this is at work or at leisure. With our everyday creativity, we adapt flexibly, we improvise, and we try different options, whether we are raising our child, counseling a friend, fixing our home, or planning a fundraising event' (2007).

While the inclusion of everyday creativity as one aspect of creativity is clearly important in order to provide a more nuanced and complete approach to creativity, the reduction of creative magnitude to two opposite poles of creativity still seems crude. Thus, though acknowledging that this kind of dichotomy is not uncommon within many areas of research, Kaufman and Beghetto recently suggested the use of two complementary facets of creative magnitude: *mini-c* and *pro-c* (2009). Mini-c refers to 'the personal … and developmental … aspects of creativity', while pro-c accounts for creativity manifested by, for example, the 'accomplished jazz musician who makes a living playing jazz (but clearly is no John Coltrane)' and thus distinguishing him from 'the high school jazz student who plays (passable) jazz in school concerts and the occasional birthday party, wedding, or family gathering'. Pro-c might be characterized as 'professional creativity' (Kaufman and Beghetto, 2009).

Big-C

Big-C creativity has the benefit of being rather unambiguous, and could therefore be said to have high *face validity*. Face validity generally refers to the appropriateness or relevance of a psychological test (Holden, 2010). Test items with high face validity generally also tend to be more technically valid, than items with lower face validity. Three components are important for face validity. First, face validity does not necessarily rest on the opinions of experts, but rather on the opinion of test takers, who may know very little about the domain investigated. Second, face validity is based on the obviousness of the test. This aspect clearly is evident in the use of genius and their works as grounds for assessment of creativity. Third, the context for which a test is assessed is important for face validity. This component highlights the temporal aspects of genius, where the definition of genius may well change over time.

Contemporary researchers have attempted to address big-C in for example important historiometric work by Dean Simonton, who defines historiometry as 'a scientific discipline in which nomothetic hypotheses about human behaviour are tested by applying quantitative analyses to data concerning historical individuals' (1984a). While the data in this type of research are archival and without randomization, the methods used are powerful and often allow accounting for potential bias (Runco, 2004).

Pro-c

Pro-c creativity refers to the category of individuals who are professional creators, but have not reached outstanding status (Kaufman and Beghetto, 2009). A good example of the need for this category is how to otherwise assess contemporary artists, such as Francis Bacon, Jean-Michel Basquiat, Louise Bourgeois, and even less known but nevertheless prominent painters, when comparing them to Leonardo da Vinci, Rembrandt, and Pablo Picasso. It may take decades to actually consider the impact of any certain artist. Conversely, some achievements that seem revolutionary may turn out to be a blind alley. There are many examples of once conspicuous but in retrospect murky achievements across most disciplines; consider, for example, the *science* of phrenology. Indeed, the definition of big-C almost necessitates a posthumous evaluation. Consequently, the concept of big-C is generally inadequate in real-world, practical situations. Nonetheless, it is interesting to note many posthumous evaluations are similar to those received during one's lifetime (Simonton, 1998). This led Kaufman and Beghetto to propose the term *pro-c*, as 'representing the developmental and effortful progression beyond little-c (but which has not yet attained big-C status)' (Kaufman and Beghetto, 2009). Kaufman and Beghetto maintain that their definition denotes everyone with professional-level expertise in any creative area. The concept of pro-c is in line with theories holding that the acquisition of expertise is necessary for creative expression (Ericsson et al., 2007). This framework pertains that prominent creators generally require 10 years of deliberate work within a domain to attain status of international expertise (Kaufman and Beghetto, 2009). In essence, pro-c does not denote big-C achievements, but rather acknowledges a solid, professional creative impact.

Little-c

Research in little-c creativity is more directed at creative everyday activities, in which laypersons can participate habitually (Richards, 2007). Studies on little-c tend to illustrate how *creative potential* is widely distributed (Runco, 2005; Runco and Richards, 1997). Research in this area may include inquiries of layperson perceptions on creativity. These generally tend to downplay analytical skills, and emphasize aspects such as unconventionality, inquisitiveness, imagination, and freedom (Kaufman and Beghetto, 2009). The standard definition of creativity, as suggested by Plucker et al. (2004); that 'Creativity is the interaction among aptitude, process, and environment by which an individual or group produces a perceptible product that is both novel and useful as defined within a social context', can be claimed to accommodate mainly for little-c. In big-C, the different aspects suggested for creativity in the standard definition are taken for granted, but the accreditation as big-C more generally relates to the impact it has had on a field. Importantly, the inclusion of little-c in creativity research has been important in dealing with some common misconceptions about creativity (Plucker et al., 2004): for example, understanding that not only certain individuals are creative but rather that creativity plays an important part in all people's lives. This is also reflected in the more nuanced approach that the question of the mad genius link has witnessed following the development of creativity research (see Chapter 6).

Mini-c

To further stress the developmental aspects of creativity, mini-c is suggested as 'the novel and personally meaningful interpretation of experiences, actions, and events' (Kaufman and Beghetto, 2009; Vygotsky, 2004). It further aligns with similar descriptions of 'personal creativity' (Runco, 1996, 2005). The concept is contingent on the Vygotskian hypotheses of cognitive and creative development arguing for all individuals having a creative potential beginning with an 'internalization or appropriation of cultural tools and social interaction. Internalization is not just copying but rather a transformation or reorganization of incoming information and mental structures based on the individual's characteristics and existing knowledge' (Kaufman and Beghetto, 2009; Moran and John-Steiner, 2003).

The benefit of introducing mini-c becomes evident when considering the creative insights of elementary or high school students. Essentially, mini-c facilitates a level of specificity ensuring that the creative potential of children is encouraged, and highlights the intrapersonal, and more process-related aspects of creativity. The creative mind of a novice, characterized by for example openness to new experiences, seems to be fundamental for most creators (Richards, 2007). It embodies the germinal, creative interpretations that all creators make, which later can develop into admired creations.

Creative magnitude in relation to psychopathology

As discussed in the previous chapter, Lombroso suggested that Galton made a fundamental flaw in confusing, talent (pro-c?) and genius, two different aspects of creative achievement (Galton, 1869; Lombroso, 1891). Lombroso's opinion was that geniuses were characterized by their severe psychopathology, whereas those with less severe psychopathologies were disdained by Lombroso, and referred to as 'mattoids' (Lombroso, 1891). The difference between talent and genius was also stressed by Lange-Eichbaum, who stated that 'talent' may have hereditary factors, whereas 'geniuses' are defined within a social context (1928; Lange-Eichbaum and Paul, 1931). Often these two go hand in hand, but he suggested not always necessarily so. Again, Juda proposed that the difference may be more of a quantitative, rather than qualitative, difference (1949). Her sub-analysis of more ordinary artists and scientists suggested that these demonstrated frequencies of psychopathology in between those highly gifted and the average population.

Contemporary research on the mad genius link has continued down the different paths of creative magnitude, and creativity research in general has increasingly directed focus on other aspects of creative achievement than merely those of geniuses. One major importance of distinguishing these two aspects is the opportunity to address more *subjective* aspects of creativity, which is more often addressed in research on little-c and mini-c, than in research on big-C (Kozbelt et al., 2010). Stein in 1953 stated that previous research mainly aiming at big-C had made investigators miss 'a necessary distinction between the creative product and the creative experience' (Stein, 1953). Focusing one-sidedly on big-C could result in bias, and the risk of excluding aspects such as creative potential (Kozbelt et al., 2010; Runco, 2007b). This is an important observation that has a major bearing on the interpretation of the mad genius link. As is evident in Chapter 6, where more recent studies on the association of creativity and psychopathology are reviewed, results suggest that patients with psychiatric disorder may well demonstrate creative potential that is not fulfilled owing to the debilitating consequences of the psychiatric disorder suffered.

To conclude on creative magnitude, Kozbelt et al. affirm the benefits of this differentiation, but also raise a more general critique, saying that (2010): 'Using these four categories [big-C, pro-c, little-c, and mini-c] in comparing theories can be helpful in highlighting the similarities and differences in the focus and scope of creativity theories. Such categories may also be helpful for considering future directions and potential connections, as well as highlighting the limitations of theories. However, the use of categories to classify creative phenomena (no matter how precise or flexible) is always limited, potentially obscuring as much as clarifying the nature of creativity.'

The four Ps

Person

An often used approach to deal with the plethora of attempts to disentangle creativity is the separation of creative studies into those directed at person, process, product or press, as suggested by Rhodes (1987). Studies on person involve, among others, research on personality traits, for which there has been a considerable amount of research (Runco, 2004). Creative individuals are suggested to have broad interests, high energy, value aesthetic qualities and autonomy, while demonstrating self-confidence and a firm sense of self as creative (Barron and Harrington, 1981). They are often considered 'contrarians' (Runco, 2007a, p. 292). The question whether there are general traits for creativity irrespective of type of creative expression (Figure 4.1), or if creative traits are domain specific (e.g., art and science) is generally also addressed in studies of person (Kaufman et al., 2009).

Motivation

Studies on person also tap into motivational research (Hennessy, 2010), a perspective on creativity which is highly relevant for the mad genius question. For example, the suggested link between bipolar disorder and high achievements have been proposed to be mediated through alterations in the *Behaviour activating system* (BAS), which is a construct in Gray's theory of personality (Gray, 1981). BAS combines several facets of motivational behaviour, e.g., focusing on reward and reward-related goals, and persistent efforts in reaching goals after preliminary success. It has been put forward that patients with bipolar disorder as well as those at risk of developing the disorder have an increased sensitivity of the BAS (Johnson et al., 2012). Prospective studies affirm that BAS sensitivity is related to the onset of bipolar disorder; the shift from cyclothymia to bipolar II disorder, the shift from bipolar II disorder to bipolar I disorder, and a more severe course of mania among those diagnosed with bipolar I disorder (Johnson et al., 2012).

Nevertheless, motivation can be framed at the concourse of state and trait (Runco, 2004). Motivation is related to mood as much as to personality. Still, it makes sense to consider the tendency to follow intrinsic

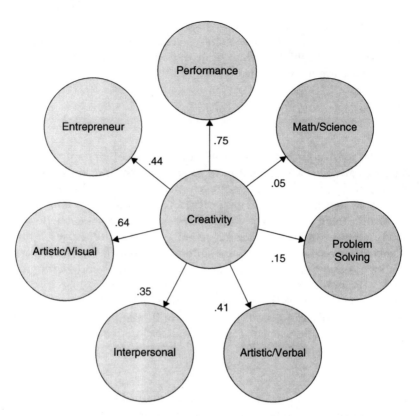

Figure 4.1   Creativity is suggested to depend on an over-arching general factor as well as seven domain specific areas of creative performance.
Source: Kaufman et al., 2009.

interests as a trait, not least considering that tasks that are intrinsically motivated tend to be free from the extrinsic evaluations (Stohs, 1992). This would make the choice of pursuing creative endeavours more contingent on personality than external factors.

Process

Research focused on the creative process is generally directed at understanding the mental processes underlying creative endeavours (Kozbelt et al., 2010). Studies may describe stages in the creative process (Wallas, 1926), and more recently be focused on cognitive aspects of creativity (Kozbelt et al., 2010).

IQ

With regards to cognitive research on creativity one very important question has been whether IQ is related to creativity or not. This inquiry was much debated at the advent of contemporary creativity research 60 years ago. One reason for this was the need for creativity research to establish itself as independent from traditional research on intelligence. Early research questioned this distinction (Getzels and Jackson, 1962), leading some researchers to focus more on tests of divergent thinking, while also providing these tests under circumstances that were presented as games rather than as tests (Runco, 2007a; Wallach and Kogan, 1965). Results supported the suggestion that creativity is distinct from intelligence; IQ, school grades, and the convergent thinking that is a prerequisite for these is independent of divergent and other aspects of creative thinking.

It was also established that the results provided under the permissive atmosphere surrounding the test situation in early research could later be reaffirmed in a setting that was less permissive and more test-like (Wallach, 1980). Tests of ideational fluency (divergent thinking) gave individual differences that were essentially independent of intelligence regardless of whether they were administered in game-like or test-like contexts. Thus, gradually empirical support for creativity being distinguishable from general measurements of intelligence as IQ were collected, which established research on creativity as a field of research in its own (Runco, 2007a).

Importantly, tests of divergent thinking, unlike traditional measurements of IQ, also display predictive validity, given that they have been shown to be moderately associated with extracurricular activities and accomplishments of students (Wallach and Wing, 1969). This finding has been replicated repeatedly (Runco, 2007a). While acknowledging that there are differences over domains of achievement, it implies that creative thinking, measured as divergent thinking, is more relevant in real-life situations than are tests of IQ or academic tests. However, keeping this benefit in mind, divergent thinking tests are only *moderately* correlated to actual achievements, which stress the limitation of psychological tests in general. They could best be referred to as indicators of *potential*.

Threshold theory   Relevant to the discussion on creativity and intelligence as separate constructs is the threshold theory. This theory holds that creativity and intelligence are correlated up to a certain level, generally up to an IQ of 120, after which there is less or no correlation (Kim et al., 2010). However, few studies have actually affirmed this empirically. Clearly a certain amount of intelligence is necessary for creativity, but more recent studies have failed to demonstrate any correlation at all between creativity and intelligence. Consider, for example a meta-analysis performed by Kim that included data from 21 studies and 45880 participants (2005), with the mean correlation coefficient being small ($r = 0.174$). Results were interpreted as the relationship being negligible, not providing support for the threshold theory.

More recent theories of intelligence have included a wider array of abilities, e.g., the Cattell–Horn–Carroll theory, which integrates 16 broad abilities of which creativity can be envisioned as one (Kim, 2005). Given this definition of intelligence, it is more pertinent to discuss what aspect of creativity (e.g., divergent thinking) or intelligence (e.g., IQ) one is referring to when suggesting that creativity and intelligence are separate constructs.

Divergent thinking

Divergent thinking is considered as a central feature of the creative process (Runco, 2010). It is employed when faced with an open-ended assignment (e.g., 'How can you use a brick?'), and is diametrical to convergent thinking in which there is only one right answer. While divergent and convergent thinking could be envisioned as a dichotomy, it seems more likely that there is a continuum from divergent to convergent thinking.

Tests assessing divergent thinking are usually designed to tap into four different aspects: *fluency* (the total number of ideas), *originality* (the number of unusual ideas), *flexibility* (the number of different categories of ideas) and *elaboration*. While divergent thinking does not equal creative thinking, divergent thinking clearly is one component of creativity. Tests assessing divergent thinking also have some major advantages over other creativity tests. Divergent thinking tests are modifiable, and allow for training, while technical aspects of reliability and validity are acceptable (Runco, 2007a). The concept of divergent thinking is also well founded in theories of creativity.

Associative theory

One such overarching theory is *associative theory*, which stipulates that ideas are linked together. Mednick suggested that the process of creativity results from the rearrangement of already prevailing ideas into new combinations (1962). These relocations are contingent on the associative strength a given idea maintains within a hierarchy of associated ideas. The steeper the hierarchy of associations is to a given stimulus, the easier it is to present one of the strongly associated ideas and the more difficult it is to come up with a weakly associated idea. Since, according to Mednick, creative ideas are defined as those with a low chance of occurring, creative individuals are suggested to have flat associative hierarchies. This would enable them easier access to more original responses.

This associative theory for creative thinking can easily be related to schizophrenia, in which early suggestions of a *loosening of associations* in psychosis was seen as a central feature leading patients to present ideas that were connected illogically to form new original groups. Bleuler thought that in schizophrenia, 'Often ideas are only partially worked out, and fragments of ideas are connected in an illogical way to constitute a new idea. Concepts lose their completeness, seem to dispense with one or more of their essential components; indeed, in many cases they are only represented by a few truncated notions ... Thus, – the process of association often works with mere fragments of ideas and concepts. This results in associations which normal individuals will regard as incorrect, bizarre, and utterly unpredictable' (Bleuler, 1911 quoted in Doughty et al., 2009).

Analogical thinking

Yet, another common theory of creative thinking is that it is based on *analogical thinking*, where one conceptual structure is used in a new setting (Welling, 2007). The classic example here is Kekulé daydreaming and envisioning a snake biting its own tail, which resulted in the discovery of the circular structure of the benzene model, and hence of all aromatic compounds (Benfey, 1958).

Dunbar specifically investigated analogical thinking in scientists, and was able to identify three different types of analogical reasoning (Dunbar, 1995). *Local analogy* is when a scientist extracts the characteristics from one experiment to another. In *regional analogy* a whole system of relationships from a similar domain is mapped onto another domain, for example, the characteristics gathered by laboratory researchers about both phage viruses and retroviruses were mapped onto each other, that is, both being members of the superordinate category virus. Thus, in order to be able to make the regional analogy, the scientists needed to have a system of relations and mechanisms in a known domain that they could then map to another similar domain. Until they had built such a representation of the primary domain, it would not have been possible to map over the other domain. This type of analogy is suggested to be relevant when working on elaborating a theory. Finally, *long distance analogy* is used when systems come from completely different domains.

This type of analogy could explain the benefits of what has been called marginality, such as for ground-breaking ideas like Darwin's on evolution (Runco, 2007a). Darwin was marginal in the sense of professionally being outside the mainstream. In theory, long distance analogy thus could benefit from psychological traits both leading to asocial behaviour, for example, schizoid personality traits, as well as those leading to common career switches, such as ADHD related traits.

Problem solving

Lastly, creative thinking has often been seen as equal to problem solving. However, not everyone agrees with this view. Guilford held that, 'I have come to the conclusion that wherever there is a genuine problem there is some novel behavior on the part of the problem solver, hence there is some degree of creativity. Thus, I am saying that all problem solving is creative. I leave the question open as to whether all creative thinking is problem solving' (Guilford, 1965 quoted in Runco, 2007a, p. 15).

Indeed, often creativity relates to creators' need of expression rather than of solving a problem. Of course, how one chooses to define something as a *problem* is also relevant. But some would say that even more than solving problems, creativity is about *finding problems*. Guilford stressed that 'sensitivity to problems' was an important aspect of creativity (1950), and there is a large literature supporting that there are individual differences in problem finding skills (Runco, 2007a).

Product

The real benefit of using the product approach in creativity research is that products can be counted. This opens up the use of powerful quantitative methodologies, as exemplified by historiometric studies (Simonton, 1984a). However, this also illustrates some of the potential limitations of the product approach. Studies in this area seldom address little-c, and obviously cannot account for creative potential. There is also the problem of distinguishing between creativity and productivity. These are, as in divergent thinking with regards to originality and fluency, correlated but not necessarily equal. In general, *originality* is the most widely acknowledged requisite for creativity (Runco, 2004). Nevertheless, while also bearing in mind that 'the best predictor of future behavior may be past creative behavior' (Colangeloa et al., 1992), some important benefits with the product approach have been incorporated in more recent inventories assessing creativity.

One of these is the Creative achievement questionnaire (CAQ), which builds on the fact that creative achievements may reflect a coming together of diverse intrapersonal and interpersonal factors (Carson et al., 2005). Such intrapersonal factors may include cognitive abilities (e.g., IQ, divergent thinking), personality traits (e.g., confidence, contrarianism), intrinsic motivation, while relevant interpersonal factors may include familial resources (e.g., ability to provide practical support), societal factors (e.g., opportunity for interaction with experts in the chosen field of creativity), and cultural considerations, such as sufficient political or economic stability.

Press

The interpersonal factors relevant for creativity are more specifically addressed in studies categorized under *press*. Press (from pressures) refers to the relationship between individuals and their environment (Rhodes, 1987). In these studies, individual differences may be seen as noise rather than what is to be investigated. Here, the focus is on general (e.g., cultural, organizational, or familial presses), and more specific (e.g., interpersonal exchanges or environmental settings) influences on creative performances (Runco, 2004).

A large part of these studies focus on social aspects (Hunter et al., 2007). They need not, however, be entirely social nor even a part of an objective experience. For example, Murray distinguished between alpha and beta pressures (1938). Alpha pressures concern more objective facets of press, while beta pressures reflect the individual's interpretation of external pressure. Simply telling people to be more original has, for example, been shown to increase the output of original ideas (Harrington, 1975). A review of studies by Hunter et al. stressed the importance of interpersonal engagement in intellectually challenging missions (2007). Other important pressures stimulating creativity are autonomy, good role models, and resources (including time) (Witt and Beorkrem, 1989). Conversely, lack of autonomy, respect, and resources as well as competition and time pressure has been found to constrain creativity (Runco, 2004). The latter do not inevitably constrain creativity, however, but should rather be seen as *potential* inhibitors. As previously suggested by Murray, there are alpha and beta pressures; one being objective and one being subjective (1938).

Competition serves as a good example for this, considering that it may both stimulate and inhibit creativity depending on the individual's interpretation (Runco, 2004). A recent study by Akinola and Mendez, takes this notion even further by adding a biological marker as possibly mediating an underlying trait interacting with external criticism (2008). The authors recruited 96 young adults (65 females) and assessed baseline levels of an adrenal steroid (dehydroepiandrosterone-sulfate, or DHEAS), previously linked to depression, as a measure of affective vulnerability. They then randomly assigned subjects to receive social rejection or social approval following reading a text aloud. Controls similarly read aloud but were not evaluated. All three groups (rejection, approval, controls) then completed artistic collages, which were upon completion evaluated by artists to assess creativity. Results confirmed a person-by-situation interaction. Social rejection was correlated to greater artistic creativity; however, the interaction between affective vulnerability (i.e., lower baseline DHEAS) and condition was significant, suggesting that situational triggers of negative affect (rejection) were especially influential among those lower in DHEAS, which resulted in the most creative products. Thus, providing support for an interaction between a biological component (person) and social pressures to artistic creativity.

An integrative model of creativity

Based on personality, process, product, and press, a number of different theories on creativity have been developed stressing these aspects of creativity to a varying degree (Kozbelt et al., 2010). Researchers have also been inspired by evolutionary biology in an attempt to address the formation of new ideas. One of these evolutionary informed theories essentially includes all Ps; person, process, product and press. This is the *Darwinian model of creativity* by Simonton (Simonton, 1984a, 1999b, 2003). In this model, aspects of person and potential is covered by addressing dispositional and developmental characteristics specifically related to the actualization of creative achievements from promising potential. The creative process is integrated by adopting a two-stage model, in which the ideational phase is outside of consciousness resulting from a blind combination of ideas generating new ideas, some of which are selected cognitively and then consciously elaborated into creative products. This creative process thus mimics biological evolution in that there is a constant flux of varying ideas, which is subsequently exposed to a selection process in which some ideas are elaborated into creative products, and these are then finally judged and again selected by society. This model essentially rests on four variables to account for creative achievements; creative potential, career duration, ideation rate, and elaboration rate (Kozbelt et al., 2010). Simonton has used historiometric investigations to provide extensive empirical support for the theory (Simonton, 1977a, 1977b, 1984a, 1985, 1988a, 1988b, 1991a, 1991b, 1997, 1998, 1999a, 1999b, 2000, 2003).

Evolution

The Darwinian model of creativity rests on the theory of biological evolution by natural selection, which was jointly presented by Charles Darwin and Alfred Wallace in 1858, and further developed in Darwin's *On the origin of species by means of natural selection* in 1859. Biological evolution is in strict terms defined as descent with modification (Futuyma, 2009). Thus, essential for evolution is variation and selection. In that certain traits are inherited, there is a variation in their representation, and a selection of these traits; some traits will increase, whereas others will decrease. The definition includes both large scale (origin of species) and small scale (changes in gene frequency in a given population) evolution.

Evolution is widely seen as one of the most influential explanatory frameworks in both biological and behavioural sciences (Cziko, 1995; Dennett, 1995). Two groups of extensions can be found as a result from the theory of biological evolution (Simonton, 1999a). The *first* type of extension is mostly relevant for biology, and adjacent fields of research. By merging with Mendelian genetics, it eventually led to the formation of such disciplines as population genetics and the recent expansion of genomics. Further theorizing and inquiries in this area resulted in the introduction of the concept of sexual selection as well as the explicit extension of the theory to elucidate the evolution of the *human species*.

Sexual selection refers to one aspect of natural selection (Campbell, 1972; Darwin, 1859, 1871; Futuyma, 2009). More specifically, it reflects an animal's ability to court and reproduce with a mate. It causes many organisms to exhibit extreme traits and behaviours, such as the elaborate tails in male peacocks, and courtship behaviour in fruit flies (Spieth, 1974). Sexual selection is powerful enough to result in traits that are harmful to the individual's survival (Zehavi and Zahavi, 1997). For example, the conspicuous tail feathers of male peacocks are likely to attract both predators as well as female peacocks. The idea of sexual selection is of major importance in more recent theories addressing the suggested association between creativity and psychopathology. This is because, some researchers have suggested, that creativity in humans is under positive sexual selection, and the capacity for creativity would thus have formed the human species throughout evolution (Miller, 2000).

The *second* type of extension that resulted from the application of evolutionary theory is that this theory provided a framework that could be generalized to all developmental or historical processes resulting from spontaneously generated variations under selection pressures (Cziko, 1995; Dennett, 1995; Simonton, 1999a). One of the earliest such *long distance analogical* applications was the now discredited Social

Darwinism (Leonard, 2009), however, other examples have received more scientific creditability (Edelman, 1987; Soderqvist, 1994).

Most interesting for the topic of this book is the application of evolutionary thinking within behavioural sciences. Evolutionary epistemologists (Campbell, 1974), argue that the cultural history of scientific knowledge is governed by the same principles that guide the natural history of biological adaptations (Simonton, 1999a). A multitude of variations of ideas first thrive, and then a few of these are selected for and retained by the sociocultural system. In science, these are the ideas that avoid extinction by Popperian falsification (Popper, 2002).

The obvious question then, is how ideas are generated in the first place? Simonton argues that it is reasonable to assume that these ideas are generated through 'a cognitive variation-selection process that occurs within the individual brain' (1999a). His theory is developed from ideas initially purported by Donald Campbell (1960), a committed proponent of evolutionary epistemology (1974).

Blind variation and selective retention

The starting point for Campbell is that the same fundamental non-teleological aspect of variation in biological evolution also applies to the creative process. He therefore named his model the blind variation and selective retention theory of creativity. The use of 'blind' was to stress the lack of foresight in the production of initial ideas. In the seminal 1960 article he says, 'real gains must have been the products of explorations going beyond the limits of foresight or prescience, and in this sense blind. In the instances of such real gains, the successful explorations were in origin as blind as those which failed. The difference between the successful and unsuccessful was due to the nature of the environment encountered, representing discovered wisdom about that environment' (Campbell, 1960). Simonton likens this outlook to when a radar systematically sweeps the skies, acting according to the principle of blindness, since it is not being guided by any *a priori* ideas about where an airplane or missile is expected to be found. However, Simonton also stresses that it is important to acknowledge that variations *need not* be totally random in the sense of demonstrating equal probability for all conceivable alternatives. It is simply suggested that the probability distribution of potential variations need not closely correspond to the probability distribution describing the variations that will actually prove successful.

This again is completely analogous to what happens in biological evolution. For example, since genes, made up of deoxyribonucleic acid

(DNA), are densely packed into chromosomes, this means that certain genetic recombinations will be more likely than others. However, these likelihoods do not necessarily reflect that certain genotypes would warrant greater reproductive fitness in the offspring. It is merely a constraint put on one of the mechanisms underlying genetic variation.

In fact, Campbell did not dismiss the prospect that some variations might be excluded on *a priori* grounds. He merely suggested that the application of such criteria depends on the previous acquisition of knowledge through a blind-variation and selective-retention process (E. Stein and Lipton, 1989). Simonton argues that this *a priori* knowledge is the result of three diverse Darwinian paths. The *first* path is by biological evolution establishing the neurological basis for human information processing. The *second* path is through individuals' trial-and-error learning, and the *third* path is social learning brought about by modelling and instruction from other individuals who themselves acquired this knowledge through trial-and-error learning (Simonton, 1999a). Under certain circumstances, the accumulation from these three paths may result in one particular activity being selected for. However, this would from a creativity perspective be the very occasions when creativity is no longer necessary.

Campbell cites personal experiences of known creators in support of his theory, such as the mathematical innovator Henri Poincaré whose experience was that (Poincaré and Halsted, 1913), '"all the combinations would be formed in consequence of the automatism of the subliminal self, but only the interesting ones would break into the domain of consciousness. And this is still very mysterious. What is the cause that, among the thousand products of our unconscious activity, some are called to pass the threshold, while others remain below? Is it a simple chance which confers this privilege? Evidently not; among all the stimuli of our senses, for example, only the most intense fix our attention, unless it has been drawn to them by other causes. More generally the privileged unconscious phenomena, those susceptible of becoming conscious, are those which, directly or indirectly, affect most profoundly our emotional sensibility ... we reach the following conclusion: The useful combinations are precisely the most beautiful, I mean those best able to charm this special sensibility that all mathematicians know, but of which the profane are so ignorant as often to be tempted to smile at it"' (Campbell, 1960).

Conferring that this type of support lacks scientific rigor, Simonton has embarked on extensive historiometric investigations to further support these ideas (Simonton, 1984a, 1999b, 2003). Including his own research, Simonton identifies three separate sources of support for the Darwinian theory of creativity. These are: experimental, psychometric, and historiometric support (Simonton, 1999a).

With regards to *experimental* support, Simonton argues both laboratory studies in human creativity as well as computer simulations of creativity in defence of the Darwinian theory of creativity. Laboratory studies in human creativity often have resorted to studies of insightful solutions (Sternberg and Davidson, 1995). Many of these studies have suggested that in order to solve a problem it is necessary to be exposed to all sorts of extraneous stimuli, both external (e.g., every day as well as professional activities) and internal (retrieved memories, chains of associative thought), which are continuously priming different aspects of the mnemonic and semantic networks during the incubation phase preceding insight (Simonton, 1999a). It is suggested that it is during this period that the mind is engaged in a blind-variation process, where the extraneous stimuli enables new conceptions to appear irrelevant to the problem at hand. This independence is essential given that the most obvious ways to solve a problem would most likely already be at hand. There is an excess of historical examples highlighting this phenomena, starting with the classic example of Archimedes in the bathtub. This would also explain the benefits seen among highly creative persons of having the tendency to engage in multiple problems simultaneously, and frequently switching topics when an obstacle seemingly stalemates a particular task (Root-Bernstein et al., 1993; Simonton, 1999a).

While most of computer simulations of creative thinking have sprung from the problem-solving approach, with 'step-by-step instructions that would lead to the solution with the absolute force of logic' (Simonton, 1999a), newer systems have allowed the development of genetic and evolutionary algorithms (GEAs) and genetic programming (Ahn, 2006; Bäck, 1996). GEAs have an enviable success record in solving real-life problems, although they still seem to lack practical applications to a large extent (Ahn, 2006). Specifically of relevance for theories of scientific creativity, however, they have for example been able to remake certain key discoveries, such as Kepler's third law of planetary motion (Koza, 1992).

Simonton also puts forth *psychometric* support for evolutionary informed theories of creativity (1999a). Thus he argues that both creativity tests and personality tests are in favour of a Darwinian perspective of creativity. For example, both Guildford's idea of a distinction between convergent and divergent thinking (1950), and Mednick's idea of highly creative individuals possessing a flat hierarchy of associations are in support of a variation-selection model (1962).

Simonton considers domain specific differences both with regards to actual testing of divergent thinking, but more importantly to the degree that a domain is reliant on, e.g, originality. For example, artistic creativity tends to be more dependent on originality and thus require a more remote approach in ideation compared to scientific creativity which is generally likely more constrained and subjected to methodological standards (Kuhn, 1962). Of course within a domain there may also be differences. Those, for example involved in what Kuhn termed *normal science* most likely do not exhibit as far-reaching generation of ideas as do those launching scientific revolutions (Simonton, 1999a).

This differentiation between the artistic and scientific domains gets even more important in relation to *personality* aspects of creativity supporting the Darwinian model of creativity. Here Simonton argues that the large body of research affirms a distinctive personality profile for creative individuals, which has been discussed previously in this chapter. These traits are concomitant on the basic assumption of the evolutionary perspective on creativity, suggesting that creative traits are those resulting in 'ideas being both numerous and diverse' (Simonton, 1999a). Therefore creative individuals tend to be 'independent, nonconformist, unconventional, even bohemian' (Simonton, 1999a), while exhibiting wide interests, openness to new experiences, and boldness.

Importantly, this would also provide an explanation for the alleged association between creativity and psychopathology (Simonton, 1999a, 1999b). According to Simonton (1999a), if 'incapacitating mental breakdowns are avoided, psychopathological symptoms can facilitate Darwinian creativity by increasing the number and scope of variations generated', since these individuals 'do not feel the inhibiting necessity of forcing their crazy hunches to conform to social and disciplinary conventions. This is an ideal situation for the production of ideational mutations'. Similarly, this would mean that due to 'the degree of variation varies across distinct domains of creativity, the expected personality profiles should follow suit. For example, artistic creators should exhibit higher levels of psychopathology than do scientific creators' (Simonton, 1999a). As has already been discussed in the previous chapter on Juda's findings (Juda, 1949), there is some support for this latter suggestion. More recent studies, including those performed by us (Kyaga et al., 2013; Kyaga et al., 2011), have also asserted a differentiation with regards to psychopathology in the artistic and scientific domains, respectively.

Simonton's final category of support for the Darwinian model of creativity is through *historiometric* evidence, where he himself has contributed with much important work (1977a, 1977b, 1984a, 1985, 1988a, 1988b,

1991a, 1991b, 1997, 1998, 1999a, 1999b, 2000, 2003). Corroborating evidence from talent development, professional careers, stylistic change, and the sociocultural environment are all adhered to in order to substantiate the evolutionary framework for creativity (Simonton, 1999a).

With regards to *talent development*, Simonton stresses the necessity of acquiring expertise essential to make a contribution to the creative domain at hand. Given that this has been argued to take about a decade of intense studies and practice (Ericsson et al., 1993; Simon and Chase, 1973; Simonton, 1997), the benefit of early acquisition is obvious. However, even though formal training may be necessary to provide the basic expertise necessary to provide a field with serious contributions, too much formal training may also constrain creativity (Simonton, 1999a). It is therefore not surprising that many of the most innovative ideas have been harvested by individuals who had their formal training in other domains than the one contributed to (Kuhn, 1962; Simonton, 1984b).

Simonton's investigations of the *professional careers* of highly gifted individuals have also provided important insights that can be seen in the light of the Darwinian perspective on creativity. For example, quite other than would maybe have been expected there seems to be a consistent relation between quantity and quality (Simonton, 1984a). Those who are most productive will have the most fruitful works, but they have also been found to have created the highest amount of work in vain. In addition, the ratio seems to hold across careers although the total quantity produced clearly varies for any individual. There is thus an *equal-odds rule* (Simonton, 1997), dictating that the appearance of what is considered quality is generally a consequence of quantity. Importantly, because of this principle creative individuals are generally not able to increase their capacity for identifying quality, but, rather since the variation process is blind, good and bad ideas appear randomly over their careers (Simonton, 1977a, 1984a, 1985, 1997). This could possibly provide another explanation for historical findings of a temporal association between creative achievements and mania in patients with bipolar disorder (Weisberg, 1994). In mania, ideation is increased (Goodwin and Jamison, 2007). Simonton also provides intriguing arguments of the Darwinian model of creativity suggested by the dramatic shifts in artistic *styles* as well in the importance of *historical and cultural environmental factors* influencing creativity (Simonton, 1999a). Essentially these arguments are based on factors stimulating a higher degree of variation in ideation.

Simonton also addresses some of the main criticisms raised for his model; for example the occurrence of multiple similar discoveries suggestive of sociocultural factors more relevant than individual factors in discoveries, individual volition and the development of domain expertise as undermining the argument for a blind variation process, and most importantly for the alleged association between creativity and psychopathology: that creativity relies on human reason (Simonton, 1999a).

In fact all of these counter-arguments can be met within the evolutionary model of creativity, for multiple similar discoveries do not contradict a blind variation process underlying creativity any more than do the multiple appearances of wings to biological evolution. The importance of human volition, a difficult concept in its own sense (Haggard, 2008), is contradicted among others by the findings supporting the equal-odds rule (Simonton, 1997).

Similarly, the relevance of acquiring expertise in a specific domain could be seen as counterintuitive to the idea of blind variation generating ideas (Ericsson et al., 1993; Simon and Chase, 1973; Simonton, 1997). However, while there are clearly domains of performance where expertise can be gathered, such as sports, games, and music (Ericsson et al., 1993), Simonton argues for some fundamental differences between these areas and other domains more strongly characterized by creativity (Simonton, 1999a). First, the former may exhibit more clearly defined criteria of success that can be closely monitored, and second truly creative domains do not demonstrate a simple linear relationship, where for instance simply running faster or winning a board of chess is always better. Creative achievements more often are characterized by striking just the right balance of originality, thus exhibiting more of an inverted U-shaped relationship in relation to success.

A multitude of different cultural factors may decide how this balance is defined. For this reason it is also questionable if the human mind is equipped to integrate all of these different aspects in order to strike the right balance. It is true though that some creative activities may be dictated by some kind of expertise. For example, the dramaturgy of many Hollywood stories may work in capturing ticket buyers, but does not necessarily implicate them as being truly creative. As has been discussed previously, there is the need to acquire fundamental domain knowledge in order to contribute to the field (Ericsson et al., 1993; Simon and Chase, 1973; Simonton, 1997), but once this knowledge is gathered there is the need for true originality, contends Simonton (Simonton, 1999a, 2006).

This is where he makes his last argument. The idea that creativity relies on blind variation is counter to major schools of creativity as problem solving arguing for it to be the 'straightforward application of conscious, logical, and deliberate analysis' (Simonton, 1999a). Although this idea of *human rationality* underlying creativity could be seen as incompatible with ideas generated by chance, it actually is not. Rather, Simonton argues that simple problems, such as the query $2 + 2 = ?$, and others may be reliant on memory retrieval alone or some other aspect of human rationality. Thus, in conscious problem solving there is no need for a blind variation-selection process, but as problems get more novel and increasingly complicated the individual has no other alternative than to resort to a combinatory process relying on random variation (Simonton, 1999a). As reviewed in Chapter 2 on the historical background of creativity, human rationality in relation to creativity is a recurring topic underlying the continuous debate on the mad genius link.

Simonton's model has been further questioned on both theoretical and empirical grounds (Kozbelt et al., 2010). Gabora suggested that the basic idea of Darwinian variation and selection is not feasible in creative thinking, 'since each thought contributes to the context in which the next is evaluated, never do the two thoughts undergo the same "selective pressure"' (Gabora, 2005). She holds that each new idea reflects both physical and social context, and that rather than the generation of discrete ideas constituting a 'hotbed' of competing ideas that are selected for, it is more parsimonious to view the generation of ideas as a state of potential ideas that can unfold in different ways depending on the context encountered. Every such development would be expected to increase the conceptual framework needed to provide creative achievements. If this is the case, then one would not expect the equal-odds rule to be manifested empirically. In fact, there is some support that the *hit-ratio* actually may improve also in more creative areas, such as music (Kozbelt, 2008). Galenson has suggested that the Darwinian model of creativity may be reconciled within a greater typological framework, where two different types of creators are found (2006); seekers, and finders. Whereas seekers work continuously, they may eventually manifest a more stable quality reliant on acquired expertise, while finders instead are characterized by making sudden changes in styles and radical contributions to a domain. Finders would therefore to a lesser extent rely on acquired expertise, and thus be more consistent with the Darwinian model of creativity.

In any case, Simonton's idea, greatly influenced by Campbell, of creativity as resulting from 'blind variation and selective retention' (1960), supported by extensive empirical data provides a framework for much of other different theories on creativity (Kozbelt et al., 2010; Simonton, 1999a). The model does not necessarily preclude that other mechanisms than the blind variation-selection may operate sometimes. It accepts that for certain situations deliberate, conscious thought may be best, but above all it stresses the force of spontaneously generated *variation of ideas* and the importance of *quantity* as central for truly creative achievements. Both these aspects may have important bearing on suggestions of an association between creativity and psychopathology manifested in specific psychiatric disorders mirroring these features (Kyaga et al., 2013; Kyaga et al., 2011; Thys et al., 2014a, 2014b).

Measuring creativity

History

There is a history of *mystifying* creativity and genius, which generally has not served research in creativity well (Plucker et al., 2004; Plucker and Makel, 2010). Several authors argue that it has resulted in researchers to shun away from creativity research, an area often characterized as *soft psychology* pervaded by several myths that have further strengthened this impression (Plucker et al., 2004; Plucker and Makel, 2010). Some of these myths are unmistakably related to the claimed inevitable link between genius and madness, as argued by Lombroso and others (1891). Many uninitiated hold that creativity cannot be measured, while commercialized training programmes in creativity, lacking both theoretical and empirical foundation, paired with antireductionist perspectives have emphasized aspects such as to 'get lost in a problem', and 'open to the irrational' (Kaufman et al., 2008; Plucker et al., 2004).

Actually, the assessment of creativity has a long history and measurements are supported by standard concepts of reliability and validity (Kaufman, Plucker et al., 2008; Plucker and Makel, 2010). In line with the previous discussion on the relationship between creativity and intelligence it is, however, paramount to more clearly define what aspect of creativity is actually being measured. Much of the psychometric research in the last decades on creativity has been overly centred on creative personality and divergent thinking (Plucker and Makel, 2010). The logic for this was partly political; creativity research needed to affirm its independence from established research in intelligence. More recent efforts of measuring creativity has included other aspects than personality and divergent thinking, while attempts at advancing established measurements in, for example, divergent thinking by developing scoring and interpretation, have also been made (Kaufman, Plucker et al., 2008). There are now literally hundreds of different tests assessing various aspects of creativity (Kaufman, Plucker et al., 2008; Plucker and Makel, 2010). Below are a few of them presented according to the framework of the four Ps.

Measuring the creative person

Research in personality traits related to creative achievements has a long and productive history. Some of the seminal studies were made during the decades following Guilford's speech in 1950 at the Institute of Personality Assessment and Research (IPAR) (Barron, 1970; Barron and Parisi, 1976; Gough, 1979; Helson, 1999; Mackinnon, 1965). Personality is defined as a 'pattern of characteristic thoughts, feelings, and behaviours that distinguishes one person from another and that persists over time and situation' (Phares, 1991, p.4). Studies have generally affirmed that personality characteristics of creative individuals include awareness of creative abilities, originality, independence, risk taking, personal energy, curiosity, humour, attraction to complexity and novelty, artistic sense, open-mindedness, need for privacy, and heightened perception, among others (Plucker and Makel, 2010).

Studies in personality traits indicative of creative potential also early suggested domain differences (Runco, 2007a). Feist performed a meta-analysis, in which he included most previous studies of personality traits in artists and scientists, comparing artists vs. nonartists, scientists vs. nonscientists, and finally creative scientists vs. less creative scientists (1998). He categorized reported traits according to the Five factor model (FFM) (R.R. McCrae and John, 1992), which is the current dominating model for personality research (Ewen, 1997; Runco, 2007a).

This FFM has considerable empirical support, and is based on factor analysis asserting the five traits: openness to experience, conscientiousness, extraversion, agreeableness and neuroticism (1992). These traits are referred to as the Big five. In general studies affirm an association between *openness to experience* and creativity (Dollinger et al., 2004; George and Zhou, 2001; Mackinnon, 1960; McCrae, 1987; Prabhu et al., 2008). Openness to experience denotes intellectual curiosity, aesthetic sensitivity, liberal values, and emotional differentiation (McCrae, 1987). Adjectives from the openness factor include those spanning from conventional–original, down-to-earth–imaginative, and uncreative–creative. In questionnaires, openness is measured in areas of fantasy, aesthetics, feelings, actions, ideas and values. These components reflect an interest in experiences for their own sake. Individuals, who are low on the openness factor are more content with the familiar and have little incentive to try the new. They therefore have little motivation to be creative. Studies investigating Big five generally use the Revised NEO personality inventory (NEO PI-R), a self-report inventory with 240 items (McCrae and Costa Jr, 2010).

Feist's analysis of artists vs. nonartists included 4397 individuals; the analysis of scientists vs. nonscientists included 4852 individuals, whereas the analysis of creative vs. less creative scientists included 3918 individuals (Feist, 1998). He also used other personality models based on factor analysis, such as the Sixteen personality factor questionnaire (16-PF) (Cattell et al.), and the Eysenck personality questionnaire (EPQ) with three factors (Eysenck, 1975). Feist concluded that the 'most striking outcome of the meta-analysis was that regardless of what measure or taxonomy was to assess personality or creativity, a consistent and clear portrait of the creative personality in science and art has emerged: Creative people are more autonomous, introverted, open to new experiences, norm-doubting, self-confident, self-accepting, driven, ambitious, dominant, hostile, and impulsive. Out of these, the largest effects sizes are on openness, [low] conscientiousness, self-acceptance, hostility, and impulsivity' (Feist, 1998). Feist's findings also revealed differences between artists and scientist. Artists were characterized more by emotional instability and the rejection of norms than were scientists. There were also differences within the group of scientists; results suggested that less creative scientists were more conscientious, conventional, and closed-minded. These results are interesting in light of the earlier discussion related to scientists within *normal science* not exhibiting as far-reaching ideas as do those initiating scientific revolutions (Kuhn, 1962; Simonton, 1999a).

The use of EPQ as a framework for Feist's meta-analysis also provided interesting results with regards to the topic of this book (Figure 4.2). Both artists and scientists demonstrated increases in the psychoticism factor, but differences with regards to the other two (extraversion and neuroticism). Psychoticism, according to Eysenck, is conceptualized as a continuum of liability to psychosis (1975, 1981; Eysenck and Eysenck, 1976). Thus, schizophrenia and to some extent bipolar disorder is viewed as being different only in degree, rather than qualitatively, from the average population (Eysenck and Eysenck, 1976).

Measuring the creative process

Divergent thinking

Measurement of creativity has to a large extent focused on aspects of divergent thinking (Kaufman, Plucker et al., 2008; Plucker and Makel, 2010). Tests assessing divergent thinking are usually designed to tap into the four different aspects: *fluency* (the total number of ideas),

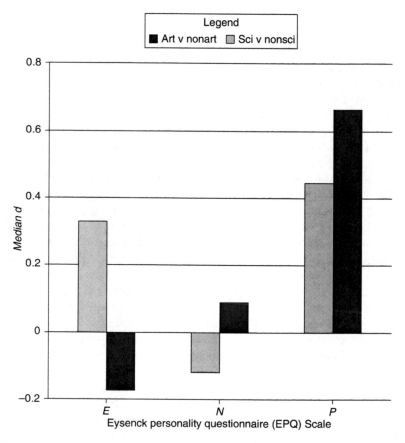

Figure 4.2   Meta-analysis of personality traits comparing artists and scientists.
Note: Both artists and scientists demonstrated increases in the psychoticism factor, but differences with regards to the other two (extraversion and neuroticism).
Source: Feist, 1998. Reprinted by permission of SAGE Publications.

originality (the number of unusual ideas), *flexibility* (the number of different categories of ideas) and *elaboration*. However, these tests generally emphasize fluency (Plucker and Makel, 2010). Tests in divergent thinking include the Guilford's structure of intellect (SOI) divergent-production tests (Guilford, 1967), Torrance tests of creative thinking (TTCT) (Torrance and Ball, 1984), and Wallach and Kogan's divergent thinking test (Wallach and Kogan, 1965). While these differ somewhat in content and instructions most provide verbal or visual prompts and ask for multiple responses. The responses are then categorized according to the different aspects of divergent thinking, i.e., fluency, flexibility, originality and elaboration.

The SOI battery consists of several tests assessing divergent thinking in different areas (Kaufman, Plucker et al., 2008); for example sketches [fluency]: drawing as many objects as possible using a basic figure, such as a circle; suffixes [fluency]: listing as many words as possible given a specific suffix; consequences [fluency]: listing commonly mentioned consequences for impossible event, such as people needing no sleep; utility [fluency]: list uses for common objects (e.g., brick, pencil); alternate letter group [flexibility]: given a set of letters, forming subgroups according to the figural aspects of the letters; alternate signs [originality]: drawing up to six symbols to represent a given concept; and figure production [elaboration]: adding lines to a simple figure to create a new figure. Wallach and Kogan devised a test similar to Guildford's but contended that providing them under a game-like situation made it possible to measure creativity distinctly from intelligence (Kaufman, Plucker et al., 2008). The most used test battery for divergent thinking is the TTCT based on many of the concepts included in the SOI (Kaufman, Plucker et al., 2008), e.g., a popular variant of the utility test called unusual uses test. One of the benefits with the TTCT is that administration, scoring, and score reporting of the various forms are standardized, and detailed norms were created and revised accordingly (Torrance and Ball, 1984).

Another test that was initially devised for measuring divergent thinking, is the Remote associates test (RAT) created by Mednick (Kaufman, Plucker et al., 2008; Mednick, 1968). This test is based on associative theory, assuming that more creative individuals should be able to make more remote associations than less creative individuals (Mednick, 1962). The test consists of 30 items with each item having three stimulus words, and the instruction to find a fourth word that is associated with the three stimulus words (Kaufman, Plucker et al., 2008). Mednick gives the following example (1968): wheel, electric, high. A scoring response would include: chair or wire. However, more recent research in patients with ADHD has suggested that the RAT may more accurately tap into convergent thinking, at least in this group of individuals (Howard-Jones and Murray, 2003; White and Shah, 2006). Thus, patients with ADHD demonstrated higher scores on the unusual uses test in the TTCT, but lower scores on the RAT, compared to individuals without ADHD. The associations were mediated through reduced inhibitory control.

In general, psychometric evidence for SOI, TTCT, RAT and other tests of divergent thinking is rather convincing (Cline et al., 1962; Plucker and Makel, 2010), but both predictive and discriminate validity have been questioned. Predictive validity refers to the ability of a test to predict future or past independent events, while discriminate validity affirms that the measurement of a construct is independent of other supposedly unrelated constructs. Later research has affirmed discriminant and predictive validity when using divergent thinking tests with methodological rigor and more content specific measurements (Plucker and Makel, 2010). Thus, in a reanalysis of previous data provided by Torrance, Plucker was able to demonstrate that divergent thinking test scores were three times superior IQ in predicting adult creative achievement (1999).

Recently, the Runco ideational behaviour scale (RIBS), has also been developed in order to provide a more appropriate criterion in estimating predictive validity of divergent thinking tests (Plucker and Makel, 2010). The RIBS emphasizes skill of generating ideas in real-life, and is a self-reported inventory with questions such as 'Friends ask me to help them think of ideas and solutions' (Runco, 2007a). Investigations of the psychometric aspects of the RIBS have concluded adequate reliability and validity (Runco et al., 2000), while other studies have affirmed its use in studies of predictive validity of divergent thinking tests (Plucker et al., 2006).

Measuring the creative product

With the main advantage of allowing for *counting*, the product approach has also been adhered to in measuring creativity; allowing for the use of potent quantitative procedures, as exemplified by historiometric studies (Simonton, 1984a). Two types of assessments within the creative products category will be reviewed below; the CAQ, and the Consensual assessment technique (CAT).

CAQ

In addition to measurements of personality traits and divergent thinking, inventories tapping into previous achievements have been developed on the assumption that 'the best predictor of future behavior may be past creative behavior' (Colangeloa et al., 1992). One such inventory, the CAQ, was previously discussed in this chapter. The CAQ is founded on the underlying assumption that creative achievements may reflect both intrapersonal and interpersonal factors (Carson et al., 2005). Such intrapersonal factors include cognitive abilities (e.g., IQ, divergent thinking), personality traits (e.g., confidence, contrarianism), and intrinsic motivation, while relevant interpersonal factors may include familial resources (e.g., ability to provide practical support), societal factors (e.g., opportunity for interaction with experts in the chosen field of creativity), and cultural considerations, such as sufficient political or economic stability. CAQ is a self-reporting inventory regarding arts (drama, writing, humour, music, visual arts and dance), science (invention, science and cooking) and architecture (Carson et al., 2005). Respondents answer to what amount the statements agree with their lifetime creative achievements (Plucker and Makel, 2010). These achievements in turn refer to the amount and type of achievements spawned (e.g., for music: no recognized talent, having played one or more musical instruments, having played with a recognized orchestra, having composed an original piece of music, having been critiqued in a local publication, having a composition recorded, having recordings to been sold publicly, and having been critiqued in a national publication); in turn referring to the amount of creative products generated (Carson et al., 2005). The results from the 10 creative domains can be individually assessed or summarized into a total score. CAQ was constructed to be objective, empirically valid, and easy to administer and score. The psychometric properties have been investigated by Carson et al. reporting acceptable results concerning reliability and validity (2005). Thus CAQ, with the additional benefit of being a non-profit self-report inventory, has been proposed as a favourable way of measuring creativity in contemporary science (Simonton, 2012).

CAT

The CAT is more clearly focused on the creative product, rather than the individual producing these products (Amabile, 1982). Some researchers argue that this provides a highly relevant approach in measuring creativity (Baer et al., 2004). It has even been put forward as the *gold standard* of creativity measurement, with the argument that the main motive for performing psychometrics in creativity is the potential of predicting the conception of future creative products (Plucker and Makel, 2010). But the question is, of course, what truly constitutes a creative product? Amabile suggests that a creative product is an artefact that is considered creative by appropriate observers (Amabile, 1982). In essence, she holds that the judgements of creativity should be done by *experts* with some kind of formal training and experience within the domain assessed (Amabile, 1996; Plucker and Makel, 2010). The CAT has been extensively used (Baer, 2003; Baer et al., 2004; Fodor and Carver, 2000; Hickey, 2001), and has gathered considerable support with regards to reliability (Plucker and Makel, 2010), and is partly supported by theory (Lim and Plucker, 2001). However, one important question has been related to the level of expertise in the creativity judges. In general, expert and novice judgements tend to be quite dissimilar (Plucker and Makel, 2010). For example, Kaufman et al. demonstrated clear differences in judgements of poetry when comparing experts and novices (college students) (Kaufman, Baer et al., 2008). In addition, prominent researchers have also questioned why expert opinions should be more valid than self-ratings and ratings by peers and parents not necessarily considered experts (Runco and Chand, 1994; Runco et al., 1994; Runco and Smith, 1992; Runco and Vega, 1990).

Measuring creative press

An often used assessment for creative pressures is the *KEYS: Assessing the climate for creativity* (Amabile et al., 1996). It is based on research in organizational creativity (Amabile and Gryskiewicz, 1989; Amabile et al., 1994; Plucker and Makel, 2010). KEYS contains 78 items measuring different aspects of work environment, such as perceived encouragement of creativity, autonomy, access to resources, as well as if the organization is perceived as creative and productive (Amabile et al., 1996). Psychometric assessments of KEYS have demonstrated acceptable reliability and validity (Mathisen and Einarsen, 2004). It has been widely used (Plucker and Makel, 2010), for example in studies of the effect for creative climate in companies downsizing (Amabile and Conti, 1999).

Summary

Contemporary research in creativity is under rapid development. Propelled by Guilford's assertion in 1950 of creativity being essential for human society, and his vision of research in creativity harbouring promises of great benefit for society, recent scientific investigations have advanced along some main paths. Among others, one has been the focus on more ordinary and psychometrically accessible aspects of creativity. Thus, a distinction has been made concerning creative magnitudes, abbreviated into big-C (genius) and little-c (everyday creativity), and further differentiated into pro-c (professional creativity) and mini-c (e.g., children's creativity). However, quantitative research in big-C has also been made possible through development in historiometric methodology pioneered by Simonton and others before him (Cox et al., 1926; Galton, 1869; Juda, 1949; Lange-Eichbaum, 1928; Lange-Eichbaum and Paul, 1931; Ludwig, 1995; Meehl, 1992; Quetelet and Beamish, 1839; Simonton, 1984a, 1999b).

One benefit of addressing less illustrious creative achievements (little-c) has been to emphasize the developmental aspects of creativity, to stress creative potential (Runco, 2005; Runco and Richards, 1997), while also reaching a standard definition of creativity, as suggested by Plucker et al. (Plucker et al., 2004): 'Creativity is the interaction among aptitude, process, and environment by which an individual or group produces a perceptible product that is both novel and useful as defined within a social context'. The increasing focus on other aspects than big-C in creativity research has also been important to deal with some common misconceptions about creativity (Plucker et al., 2004). For example, understanding that creative individuals are not unique but rather that creativity plays a significant part in all people's lives. It has also been reflected in more recent studies providing a more nuanced association between creativity and psychopathology. These studies are reviewed in Chapter 6.

Research in creativity is often categorized according to those studies directed at the creative personality, the creative process (e.g., divergent thinking), the creative product, or social pressures influencing creativity (Rhodes, 1987). Simonton has proposed an overall model of creativity, previously suggested by Campbell, of new ideas resulting from 'blind variation and selective retention' (1960). This model is supported by extensive empirical data, and provides a framework for much of other different theories on creativity (Kozbelt et al., 2010; Simonton, 1999a). It advocates that ideas are unconsciously generated, and then some of these are selected first through cognitive mechanisms within the individual, but then later through social pressures. This model stresses the importance of *quantity* of ideas as fundamental for truly creative achievements.

Each of the different aspects of creativity, i.e., person, process, product, and press, can be measured by different tests. Overall, these tests demonstrate acceptable standards of reliability and validity, and have in some cases been able to provide better predictive validity than more standard intelligence measurement, such as IQ (Plucker, 1999). Early studies also affirmed that creativity is independent of IQ, which established creativity research as a field in its own (Kim et al., 2010; Runco, 2007a).

The creative personality has often been assessed within the FFM, demonstrating an association between *openness to experience* and different measurements of creativity (Feist, 1998). Measurements of divergent thinking, such as SOI or the TTCT (Guilford, 1967; Torrance and Ball, 1984), have often been used to tap into the creative process.

Lastly, more recent inventories have approached the assessment of creative products and pressures, by looking into individual's previous achievements, e.g., the CAQ (Carson et al., 2005), by using panels of creativity judges to assess the inherent creativity of artefacts (Amabile, 1982), and assessing perceived aspects of work environment (Amabile et al., 1996).

5
Biological Perspectives on Creativity

Introduction

Recent years have seen a strong development of a comparably neglected aspect of research in creativity: the biological basis of creativity. This development has been manifested in an increasing number of original articles and reviews covering this area (Arden et al., 2010; Dietrich, 2004; Dietrich and Kanso, 2010; Gonen-Yaacovi et al., 2013; Runco et al., 2011). Two main areas can be identified: genetics and neurophysiology. Both these areas have seen astonishing advances in recent decades with new methodologies being used for a number of different aspects of psychology and psychiatry (Gazzaniga et al., 2009; Plomin et al., 2012).

The genetics of creativity

The genetic aspect of creativity has been investigated by two main approaches. Early attempts were directed at assessing whether creative achievements and giftedness were *inherited*. This approach was pioneered by Francis Galton (see Chapter 3), and has since been further developed into complicated models accounting for such aspects as *gene-environment interactions* and *assortative mating*, the latter referring to individuals with similar genes and traits more often tending to mate with one another than what would be expected by chance (Plomin et al., 2012). A good example of this is that individuals with *similar heights* are inclined to mate (MacDougall and Montgomerie, 2003; Stulp et al., 2013). More recent attempts at investigating the genetic underpinnings of creativity have directly assessed specific *candidate genes* through molecular genetics (Reuter et al., 2006).

The construct of heritability

Formally, *heritability* provides an estimate of the genetic proportion underlying a trait (Plomin, 2008). Traits are generally referred to as the *phenotype*, denoting the observable trait, for example eye colour or personality trait, and placed in relation to the *genotype*, which carries the hereditary information. However, heritability is also a word that is commonly used by laymen to describe that a certain feature is heritable (Stoltenberg, 1997). This vagueness in use is most likely the reason for some common misperceptions related to studies of heritability.

Heritability in its formal meaning contains an estimate of the proportion of genetic effect, ranging from 0 (no variation in phenotypic variation due to variation in genotype) to 1 (all phenotypic variation due to variation in genotype). Because many estimates of heritability of psychological traits are deduced from small cohorts, heritability studies often suffer from low power (Linney et al., 2003). The consequence of this is that estimates in heritability can vary considerably owing to *chance errors*.

Importantly, the effect size or genetic proportion of a trait refers to the amount of variance explained within a *group*. Thus, heritability does not define the phenotype of a *single individual* and does not imply genetic determinism. Instead, it reveals the genetic component of individual differences for a given trait in a population at a given time. Thus, if the influence of genes were to be altered (e.g., due to mutation or migration) or if environmental changes happened (e.g., through education), the relative impact of genes and environment, respectively, would change.

Studies of heritability often use twin and family designs, both of which have a long history dating back to Francis Galton (see Chapter 3) (1869). One of the first modern twin studies, however, was conducted by Merriman in 1924, where identical and fraternal twins were compared in an effort to estimate the genetic influence on IQ.

Twin studies rely upon the fact that monozygotic (MZ) twins are genetically identical, while fraternal (dizygotic, or DZ) share on average 50 per cent of their genomes identical by descent. Intra pair correlations of an investigated trait can then be used to calculate the genetic effect under the assumption that the difference of correlations in MZ-pairs compared to correlations in DZ-pairs corresponds to half of the genetic effect. Therefore, given that the correlation of IQ in identical and fraternal twins is, for example 0.86 and 0.60, respectively (Bouchard and McGue, 1981), then doubling the difference between these two estimates would correspond to the full genetic impact of 0.52 ($0.86 - 0.60 = 0.26$; $0.26 \times 2 = 0.52$). Thus, about half of the variance in IQ can be explained by genetic factors (heritability).

Twin studies also convey two other components: *shared environment*, affecting both twins similarly, and *unshared environment*, which is the unique environmental stimuli that meet one twin but not the other, or stimuli that affect each twin differently. Together these three components are abbreviated ACE; the genetic component (A), the shared environment (C), and the unshared environment (E).

While estimates derived from twin studies are firmly based on empirical investigations, studies of heritability are often misinterpreted. Common misconceptions are that a high heritability implies genetic determinism and that heritability conveys information about between-group differences. Though a high heritability estimate for a certain trait implies that the genetic component is important, it does not mean that the phenotype is determined once the specific genotype is known. One example of this is height, which is estimated to have a substantial heritability of 0.8 (Cole, 2000; Visscher et al., 2006). However, the increase in mean height that has occurred in many societies in the last century most likely reflects increased access to healthcare and good nutrition, i.e. changes in environment. Similarly, heritability estimates cannot be used for between-group comparisons; groups differing in height do not necessarily do so because of genetic differences.

To summarize, heritability is an important but also limited factor in genetics, allowing for an estimate of the relative impact of genes and environment on a given trait in a specific population at a given time. It directs attention at a broad array of phenotypes, where genes are likely to be important (Visscher et al., 2008).

Molecular genetic approaches

DNA

DNA (deoxyribonucleic acid) is the molecule that is responsible for heredity (Plomin, 2008). In 1953, James Watson and Francis Crick suggested a molecular structure for DNA that was able to explain both how genes coded for proteins, and how genes were replicated. The basis for the DNA molecule is two strands held together by pairs of four bases: adenine (A), thymine (T), guanine (G), and cytosine (C). The bases of each strand always pairs as A-T and G-C.

The two strands may separate, which allows for *replication*, by each strand attracting new appropriate bases (A to T, etc.) to the already existing bases, thereby forming two new double strands. In addition, a strand may be *transcribed* into a different sort of nucleic acid called *ribonucleic acid* (RNA), which in turn may be *translated* into proteins by three bases (codon) at a time of the RNA being interpreted as one of 20 specific *amino acids*. The combination of these amino acids results in the production of the different *proteins* in the body and brain. A third of all protein coding genes are expressed only in the brain.

A *gene* denotes a region of the DNA (or RNA) resulting in the production or the regulation of the production of a protein. *Genome* refers to all genes in a certain organism, while *alleles* refer to the different variants of a given gene. The genome is stored on large *chromosomes*, of which humans have 23 pairs (one from each parent). *Homozygotes* have the same allele in a given gene in these pairs, while *heterozygotes* have different alleles in these pairs.

Candidate genes

Specific *DNA-markers* has made it possible to compare, for example, patients with schizophrenia cases to healthy controls with regards to specific alleles (Sun et al., 2008). This kind of research is usually hypothesis driven in that certain *candidate genes* are investigated based on theoretical grounds. One example of this approach is studies of genes coding for proteins responsible for the function of the neurotransmitter dopamine in relation to different aspects of creativity (Murphy et al., 2013; Reuter et al., 2006; Runco et al., 2011). However, a recurring problem with the candidate gene approach has been that positive findings have been difficult to replicate (Chabris et al., 2012; Plomin, 2008). In addition, the candidate gene approach is not systematic, but rather relies on theoretical presumptions.

These limitations have gradually made investigators use a genome-wide approach in which a dense map of 500000 DNA-markers or more are investigated without necessarily directing focus towards specific genes. This approach thus calls for comprehensive correction of *multiple comparisons* to avoid chance findings. The result has been that studies using a genome-wide approach have included a great number of individuals as cases and controls. This has also made problems of *matching* evident, since systematic bias in matching of cases and controls potentially could lead to serious systematic errors (Humphreys et al., 2011). More recent research has adopted *polygenic scores* to summarize genetic effects among an ensemble of markers that do not individually achieve significance in a genome-wide association study (Dudbridge, 2013), and whole-genome sequencing; determining every base in the DNA (Sharma et al., 2014).

Review of research on the genetics of creativity

We recently systematically reviewed the literature on the genetics of creativity (Kyaga, 2014), with the objective of providing a complete overview of studies focusing or relating to genetic influences on creativity. The review was conducted using the Prisma Statement methodology, which is an established evidence-based minimum set of items for reporting in systematic reviews and meta-analyses (Moher et al., 2009). All original studies in English, including quantitative meta-analyses, were considered for inclusion. Studies were collected through the databases PubMed, the Web of Science, and PsychINFO, with additional articles added after going-over the reference lists of relevant articles. The different *study designs* in the included articles were categorized into a) family studies, b) twin studies, c) adoption studies, d) candidate gene studies, or e) other studies. Three different categories for the *definition of creativity* (category of definition) were chosen; a) eminence, b) inventory, and c) creative occupation.

Additionally, three different categories for the *quality* of the included studies were defined. High quality was defined as *valid definition of creativity, comparative study design, adequate statistical analysis and power*, and medium quality as *unvalidated measurement of creativity, comparative study design, adequate statistical analysis and power*. All other studies were defined as having low quality. For studies considered to have high quality, the study design additionally had to be explicitly aimed to address a genetic component of creativity, for example the heritability of creativity or a candidate gene approach. Findings were categorized as: positive, negative, or conflicting. Those studies labelled under conflicting findings were reporting both positive and negative findings (e.g., positive for one type of creativity measurement and negative for another).

More than half of the studies included (52 per cent) used inventories to define creativity, while 39 per cent used eminence and 9 per cent used creative occupations. With regards to study design, 55 per cent were family studies, 21 per cent twin studies, 14 per cent candidate gene studies, 5 per cent adoption studies, and 4 per cent used other study designs. About a third of the studies were considered having high quality (34 per cent), while 36 per cent were of medium quality, and 30 per cent had low quality. The number of articles included steadily increased from those published at the end of the nineteenth century, with a peak about two decades ago. Nevertheless, the number of included studies with *high quality* continues increasingly to be published today. A total of 19 studies were categorized as having high quality. Ten of these used twin design, one was an adoption study, while the others (n = 8) were candidate gene studies. Of the latter, the first was published in 2006 (Reuter et al., 2006), thus candidate gene studies were in general more contemporary than other studies reviewed.

It is possible that the included studies may reflect *publication bias* as well as selective reporting within studies. Publication bias refers to bias resulting from only certain results being published, mostly positive rather than negative findings. This is not least evident in the studies using a candidate gene approach, since all candidate gene studies on creativity to some extent reported positive results. On the other hand, the majority of these studies also reported on negative findings related to various candidate genes.

Overall, results regarding the genetics of creativity are conflicting both across and within studies of this review. Of the 56 original studies included, 48 demonstrated positive findings of familiality or a specific genetic component, 6 demonstrated conflicting results, while 2 demonstrated negative results. Thus, 86 per cent of studies demonstrated positive results, while 14 per cent demonstrated conflicting or negative results. Familiality, however, is not the same thing as a hereditary component since familiality could be due to *shared environmental* factors.

Heritability of creativity   The twin design has been accused of inflating estimates of the genetic component, since the design rests on the *equal environments assumption*. This assumption refers to the idea that MZ twin pairs and DZ twin pairs share equal environment, which has been challenged repeatedly (Plomin, 2008; Visscher et al., 2008). If MZ twins were to share more environment (e.g., treated more similar) than DZ twins, then this would result in the genetic component being overestimated. However, the equal environments assumption has been tested in several studies and seems to be reasonably stable for most traits investigated (Plomin, 2008).

Focusing on the 10 twin studies of high quality revealed that only six established positive results, while three demonstrated conflicting results and one had negative results. However, as described previously conflicting or negative findings could possibly reflect the fact that studies with these results generally were smaller. In the studies with positive results the number of included twin pairs ranged from 77 to 1618, while those with conflicting results ranged from 61 to 116, and the study with negative results included 65 twin pairs.

In high quality twin studies reporting positive results (n = 6), estimations of heritability ranged from 0.22 (Nichols, 1978) to 0.78 (Barron, 1970). It should be noted that the included studies generally measure different aspects of creativity. Estimations of heritability in high quality twins studies reporting positive results specifically using *divergent thinking* ranged from 0.22 (Nichols, 1978) to 0.43 (Grigorenko et al., 1992).

The first high-quality twin study included was published in 1932 (Carter, 1932). It collected information on vocational interests in 120 twin pairs. Intraclass correlations in, for example, being an *artist* were 0.44 for MZ twin pairs and 0.20 for DZ twin pairs, thus implying about half of the variance being explained for by genetic effects in artistic inclination. Nichols reviewed studies on artistic interests and found intraclass correlations of 0.50 for MZ twin pairs and 0.30 for DZ twin pairs, resulting in similar estimates as Carter (1978). He also found similar heritability in scientific interests; MZ twin pairs with intraclass correlation of 0.54, and DZ twin pairs of 0.29. Canter addressed creative personality and found some evidence for heritability in imaginativeness, assessed by Cattell's 16-PF (1973). However, Waller et al. later demonstrated considerable differences in intraclass correlation between MZ twin pairs and DZ twin pairs when assessing 78 twin pairs with the Creative personality scale (1993). Barron et al. investigated 61 twin pairs and demonstrated that aesthetic abilities, as measured by, for example, the Frank drawing completion test (FDCT), had substantial heritability estimates over 0.6, but that aesthetic preferences as measured by, for example, the BWAS demonstrated no evidence of heritability (Barron and Parisi, 1976). The FDCT consists of 36 unfinished drawings in which the subject is supposed to complete drawings with as many lines as he or she likes (Reznikoff et al., 1973). Protocols are scored for originality. Given that this study only included 61 twin pairs, the authors suggested that results should be considered with caution.

Reznikoff et al. in a larger study of 117 twin pairs was not able to demonstrate any considerable heritability for the FDCT or the BWAS, but reported heritability estimates at 0.56 for the RAT (see Chapter 4) (1973). Most twin studies assessing aspects of divergent thinking found differences in intraclass correlations between MZ twin pairs and DZ twin pairs indicative of heritability (Barron, 1970; Grigorenko et al., 1992; Nichols, 1978; Reznikoff et al., 1973; Vandenberg, 1967). Although Pezzullo was unable to demonstrate a genetic component in a study of 65 twin pairs using the unusual uses test of the TTCT (1971). As previously mentioned, however, this study was comparable small to other studies demonstrating varying heritability in divergent thinking.

The one *adoption study* included within the group of high quality studies demonstrated that of the adoptees in the high creativity group, 30 per cent suffered a mental illness, while this was true for 27.8 per cent of their biological parents, and only 5.3 per cent of their adoptive parents (McNeil, 1971). The authors concluded that these findings suggested that prenatal factors (e.g., genes) influenced the association between creativity and mental illness.

Candidate gene studies on creativity Candidate gene studies on creativity addressed specific genes that on theoretical basis are suggested to be associated with creativity. Most of the genes investigated have also been investigated in relation to psychiatric disorders in other studies (Schatzberg and Nemeroff, 2009).

All studies except one (Ukkola-Vuoti et al., 2013) published with a candidate gene approach demonstrated significant findings with regards to some measurement of creativity (n = 7). These studies generally all investigated different genes using diverse measurements for creativity. The results based on present findings should therefore be interpreted with caution (Chabris et al., 2012). However, initial findings of dopamine receptor D2 gene (DRD2) being related to verbal creativity, and tryptophan hydroxylase gene 1 (TPH1) being related to figural creativity can be said to have been partly replicated (Reuter et al., 2006; Runco et al., 2011). As of yet, no study has incorporated more recent genome-wide methodology on a large scale, though Ukkola-Vouti et al. used a whole-genome approach addressing copy number variations (large structural genetic alterations) in a comparable small sample of 341 individuals (2013).

Studies investigating creativity using the candidate gene approach (Table 5.1) have generally investigated genes related to the *mono-aminergic neurotransmission* or genes related more specifically to *neuronal development*. Neurotransmission is a vital process for neuronal differentiation and growth in the brain, as well as for its interneuronal communication and neuronal circuitry (Kurian et al., 2011). The monoamines are a central group of brain neurotransmitters, consisting of the catecholamines (dopamine, norepinephrine and epinephrine) and serotonin. Dopamine and serotonin play key roles in controlling movement, mood and behaviour (Egerton et al., 2009; Schatzberg and Nemeroff, 2009). Dopamine has also been implicated in mediating the creative process (Flaherty, 2005).

The first study performed using a candidate gene approach in relation to creativity was published in 2006 with 92 healthy individuals investigating the Catechol-O-methyltransferase gene (COMT VAL158MET), the DRD2 gene (TAQ IA), and the serotonergic gene TPH1 (TPH-A779C) (Reuter et al., 2006). COMT is a crucial enzyme inactivating catecholamines. A gene variant of COMT, where the amino acid methionine (MET) has been supplemented with valine (VAL) results in a 3- to 4-fold increase in COMT enzyme activity. Heterozygotes (VAL/MET genotype), have intermediate COMT activity. The lower rates of COMT activity with the MET allele leads to increased dopamine levels, with ensuing cognitive consequences. Studies have for example found the best working memory performance in carriers of the MET/MET genotype and the worst performance in carriers with the VAL/VAL genotype (Goldberg et al., 2003). The dopamine D2 receptor (DRD2) gene, coding for one of five dopamine receptors, can be homozygotes for A1 (A1A1), but this is uncommon and the different polymorphisms (variants of a gene leading to a phenotypic difference) are usually referred to as A1+ (homozygous for A1 or heterozygous), or as A1-(homozygous for A2 (A2A2)). In A1+ individuals, there is a 30–40 per cent reduction in dopamine receptor D2 density compared to A1- individuals (Ritchie and Noble, 2003). DRD2 has been implicated especially in avoidance learning (Frank and Fossella, 2011). TPH is the rate-limiting biosynthetic enzyme in the serotonin (5-HT) pathway and controls levels of 5-HT by converting tryptophan into 5-hydroxytryptophan, which is the direct precursor of 5-HT (Reuter et al., 2006). The 5-HT system plays an important role in cognitive functioning and psychiatric disorders (Reuter et al., 2006; Schatzberg and Nemeroff, 2009). It is plausible that variations in the TPH gene could contribute to low activity of the 5-HT system.

Both DRD2 and TPH1 genes, but not COMT, were associated with creativity as measured by the inventiveness scale of Berlin intelligence structure test (Reuter et al., 2006). These results were followed up by Runco et al. in 2011 on 147 healthy individuals using more standard tests of divergent thinking (verbal and figural) as well as a realistic creative problem-solving task. Results partly replicated previous findings in that TPH1, and other genes related to dopamine metabolism were implicated (though not for DRD2). Results were corrected for IQ, and suggested that the positive findings were mostly due to increased fluency (ideation), rather than originality. These results were further reanalysed to account for polygenic interactions, and to investigate specific divergent thinking tasks instead of a composite scores (M. Murphy et al., 2013). The latter meant that the DRD2 gene became significantly associated with verbal fluency.

A study by Keri is intriguing in relation to the present book, since this study demonstrated an association between a polymorphism of the Neuregulin 1 gene the CAQ and the Just suppose test of the TTCT in 200 healthy individuals (Kayser, 2013; Keri, 2009). This gene has been suggested as a risk factor for developing psychosis (Bousman et al., 2013). Neuregulin 1 protein exists in different forms, with different functions,

Table 5.1 High quality studies on genetics in creativity

Study	Objective	Definition of Creativity	Population (n)	Outcome	Comments	Findings
TWIN STUDIES						
(Carter, 1932)	Heritability	The Strong vocational interest blank	120 pairs of twins. MZ pairs (21 males, 22 females), DZ same sex pairs (22 males, 21 females). 34 DZ pairs of unlike sex.	Intraclass correlations	Intraclass correlations (rMZ, rDZ) for interest in: Artist (0.44, 0.20), Chemist (0.64, 0.39), Psychologist (0.36, 0.32), Physicist (0.65, 0.33), Mathematician (0.54, 0.27).	Positive
(Vandenberg, 1967)	Heritability	Nine divergent thinking (DT) tests: pertinent questions, different uses, social institutions, seeing deficiencies, making a plan, similar words, association, figure production, picture arrangements	91 pairs of twins. MZ pairs (67), DZ pairs (24). Data on sex not present.	Intraclass correlations	Lack of significance for a genetic factor except test: pertinent questions.	Conflicting
(Barron, 1970)	Heritability	– Adaptive flexibility (Crutchfield revision of the Gottschaldt figures) – Expressional fluency (Guilford battery) – Ideational fluency (Guilford battery) – Originality (Guilford battery) – Esthetic judgment for visual displays (BWAS)	Italian sample: 59 pairs of twins. MZ pairs (15 males, 15 females), DZ same sex pairs (14 males, 15 females). American sample: 57 pairs of twins. MZ pairs (14 males, 15 females), DZ same sex pairs (13 males, 15 females).	Intraclass correlations	– Findings are inconsistent (varying considerable depending on which sample investigated). – Visual tests generally reveal significant differences between monozygotic and dizygotic twins (h^2 0.41 in American sample and 0.78 in Italian sample), compared to verbal tests.	Conflicting

(Pezzullo, 1971)	Heritability	TTCT, verbal B unusual uses of tin cans for divergent thinking	65 pairs of twins. MZ pairs (37), DZ pairs (28). Data on sex not present.	Intraclass correlations	- Failure to demonstrate a significant genetic component in verbal divergent thinking.	Negative
(Canter, 1973)	Heritability	EPQ (40 MZ, 45 DZ), Sociability/Impulsivity Scale (40 MZ, 45 DZ), Catell's 16PF (39 MZ, 44 DZ), Fould's hostility scale (39 MZ, 44 DZ)	83 pairs of twins. MZ pairs (9 males, 30 females), DZ pairs (14 males, 30 females).	Intraclass correlations	Intraclass correlations for imaginativeness in 16PF were rMZ: 0.23 and rDZ: 0.08 overall. In females rMZ: 0.23 and rDZ: 0.11; in males: rMZ: 0.24 and rDZ: -0.04.	Positive
(Reznikoff et al., 1973)	Heritability	Battery of 11 creativity tests (Remote associates test, Franck drawing completion test, Associational fluency test and Expressional fluency test, BWAS, Alternate uses test, Possible jobs test, Plot titles test, Obscure figures test, Similes test, Quick word test)	117 pairs of twins. MZ pairs (28 males, 35 females), DZ pairs (19 males, 35 females).	Intraclass correlations	- Identical twins are more alike than fraternals on various measures of creativity. - Significant findings in Remote associates test ($H = .56$), Plot titles ($H = .21$), and similes ($H = .39$).	Positive
(Barron and Parisi, 1976)	Heritability	- The Gough-McGurk perceptual acuity test - Gottschaldt figures - Franck drawing completion test - Irwin child test of esthetic judgment - The Barron M-threshold inkblot test - BWAS - The Gough adjective check list - Expressive behavior sample	61 pairs of twins. MZ pairs (36), DZ pairs (25). Twins were approximately equally divided between male and female.	Intraclass correlations	- Perceptual and esthetic abilities appear to have substantial heritability (>.6), whereas esthetic preferences do not. - Heritability was also indicated in adjectives such as artistic, inventive, original, and independent.	Conflicting

(continued)

86

Table 5.1 Continued

(Nichols, 1978)	Heritability	Divergent thinking, science interest, artistic interest	Twin literature up to 1971 was reviewed for a variety of psychological traits (756 twin pairs). In addition analyses of two twin samples were made (850 pairs (60% MZ and 42% males) and 1618 pairs (61% MZ and 41% males), respectively).	Intraclass correlations	Intraclass correlations for rMZ, rDZ respectively; Divergent thinking (0.61, 0.50; 10 studies), Science interest (0.54, 0.29; 15 studies), Artistic interest (0.50, 0.30; 16 studies).	Positive
(Grigorenko et al., 1992)	Heritability	TTCT, verbal, form A	123 pairs of twins. MZ pairs (26 males, 34 females), DZ pairs (26 males, 37 females).	Intraclass correlations	Heritability = 0.43	Positive
(Waller et al., 1993)	Heritability	Creative personality scale of the adjective check list	78 pairs of twins. 45 pairs of reared-apart MZ, one set of reared-apart identical triplets, and 32 pairs of reared-apart DZ.	Intraclass correlations	- Intraclass correlation of monozygotic twins was 0.54. - Intraclass correlation of dizygotic twins was -0.06. - Results suggesting that creativity is an 'emergenic' trait.	Positive

ADOPTION STUDIES

Study	Design	Definition/Method	Sample	Measures	Results	Direction
(McNeil, 1971)	Genetic liability	Creative ability was defined by a committee evaluation, dividing subjects into; high-, above-average-, low-creative ability	43 adults (10 males were considered high creative) adopted by nonbiologically related families in the Copenhagen metropolitan area 1924–1947 was compared to 23 matched noncreative adoptees.	Frequencies in adoptees and their parents	– Mental illness rates in the adoptees were positively related to their creative abilities. – Mental illness rates of the biological parents were positively related to the creative abilities of the adoptees. – Mental illness rates among adoptive parents were independent of the adoptees' creative abilities. – Data were interpreted as evidence for influence of prebirth (e.g., genes, intrauterine) factors on creative ability and mental illness.	Positive

CANDIDATE GENE STUDIES

Study	Design	Definition/Method	Sample	Measures	Results	Direction
(Reuter et al., 2006)	Association	– Creativity testing using the test battery inventiveness of the Berlin intelligence structure test – Intelligence testing for fluid intelligence by Cattell's CFT-3 and crystallized intelligence by the subtest knowledge of the Structure-of-intelligence-test	92 healthy individuals (17 males, 75 females).	– Catechol-O-methyltransferase gene (COMT VAL158MET) – Dopamine D2 receptor gene (DRD2 TAQ IA) – Serotonergic gene TPH1 (TPH-A779C)	– DRD2 gene and the TPH gene were associated with creativity, explaining 9% of the variance. – COMT was not related to creativity at all. – DRD2 was related to verbal creativity and TPH1 to figural and numerical creativity.	Positive

(continued)

Table 5.1 Continued

(Schmechel, 2007)	Association	Artistic avocations (n = 189) and vocations (n = 57)	1537 (664 males, 873 females) consecutive patients at Duke University Memory Disorders Clinic.	A1AT polymorphisms	In persons with artistic avocation or vocation, AAT non-M polymorphisms are significantly increased (respectively, proportions of 44 and 40% compared to background rate of 9%; p = 0.0007).	Positive
(Keri, 2009)	Association	– IQ (Wechsler), socioeconomic status (Hollingshead four-factor index), schizotypal traits (Schizotypal personality questionnaire), CAQ, the just suppose subtest of TTCT	200 healthy individuals (101 males, 99 females)	A functional promoter polymorphism of the Neuregulin 1 gene (SNP8NRG243177/ rs6994992)	– T/T genotype associated with increases in CAQ and with all aspects of just suppose subtest. – The T/T genotype of Neuregulin 1 gene has formerly been associated with increased psychosis risk.	Positive
(Runco et al., 2011)	Association	– Divergent thinking tests (verbal and figural) – Realistic creative problem solving – Wonderlic intelligence test (for adjusting)	147 healthy individuals (49 males, 98 females).	Candidate genes (DAT1, COMT, DRD4, DRD2, TPH1)	– Verbal fluency associated to DAT1, DRD4, COMT. – Figural fluency associated to COMT, TPH1, DRD4. – Verbal originality associated to DAT, DRD4, DRD2. – Figural originality associated to DAT, DRD4. – Ratio originality/fluency in verbal or figural no association to genes. – Flexibility associated to DAT. – No association to genes in realistic problem. – Adjusting for intelligence did not ameliorate differences in genes.	Positive

(Schmechel and Edwards, 2012)	Association	Artistic avocations and vocations	3176 consecutive patients presenting to Duke University Memory Clinic (747 patients (321 males, 426 females)) and to a regional community-based Caldwell hospital neurology and memory center (2429 patients (891 males, 1538 females)).	A1AT polymorphisms	Odds ratio is 3.7 (3.0–4.5) for artistic vocation/avocation for carriers of mutation. Data present on 2885 individuals.	Positive
(Soeiro-de-Souza et al., 2012)	Association	BWAS and other neuropsychological tests	66 subjects (22 males, 44 females) with bipolar disorder (41 in manic and 25 in depressive episodes) and 78 healthy controls (39 males, 39 females).	BDNF polymorphism (Val66Met)	Manic patients with Val allele (Met−) had higher BWAS scores than Met+ carriers. This was not seen among patients in depressive episodes or among control subjects.	Positive
(M. Murphy et al., 2013)	Association	Divergent thinking tests (verbal and figural)	147 healthy individuals (49 males, 98 females).	Candidate genes (DAT1, COMT, DRD4, DRD2, TPH1)	Reanalysis of Runco et al. 2011 demonstrated both verbal fluency and verbal originality were related to significant interactions between DRD2 X DAT, DRD2 XDRD4, DAT X COMT, COMT X DRD4, DRD2 XDAT X COMT, and DRD2 X COMT XDRD4.	Positive

(continued)

Table 5.1 Continued

| | | Association | Creativity in music (composing, improvising and/or arranging music) was surveyed using a web-based questionnaire | Five extended pedigrees (n = 169 (81 males, 88 females) and unrelated subjects (n = 172 (71 males, 101 females)). | Copy number variations (CNVs) | – A deletion at 5p15.33 containing the gene ZCHHC11 was present in 48% and a duplication at 2p22.1 containing the gene GALM was present in 27% of creative family members.
– In the unrelated sample set no significant excess of large CNVs or CNV burden were detected in the creative or non-creative phenotypes. | Conflicting |
| (Ukkola-Vuoti et al., 2013) | | | | | | | |

but has generally been implicated in neuronal growth and myelination (isolating the axon of the neuron), as well as protection of dopaminergic neurons. So far these findings have not been replicated.

Another fascinating study was performed by Soiera-de-Souza et al., who investigated 66 patients with bipolar disorder, and 78 healthy controls assessed for creativity with the BWAS in relation to a gene coding for Brain-derived neurotrophic factor (BDNF) (2012). The BWAS has previously been suggested to specifically be of relevance for affective processing, making it of particular interest in assessing relationships between mood and creativity (Simeonova et al., 2005). BDNF on the other hand is an important neurotrophic factor (stimulating neuronal growth). A polymorphism substituting valine (VAL) with methionine (MET), resulting in decreased substitution of BDNF has been found to lead to impaired performance in memory, executive functions, and intelligence. The authors investigated how this polymorphism interacted with mood in patients with bipolar disorder, and found that manic patients homozygous for the VAL allele had higher BWAS scores than MET+ carriers. This relationship was not observed among patients in depressive episodes or among controls. Since mania has been postulated to encompass higher dopamine levels, the authors speculated that the increased dopamine function may interact with BDNF leading to higher creativity scores in BWAS.

Yet, another study investigated polymorphisms of the gene for serine protease inhibitor alpha-1-antitrypsin (A1AT) (Schmechel, 2007; Schmechel and Edwards, 2012). A1AT is a protein released in response to inflammation and trauma. These were four-fold increases in an unusual polymorphism of the A1AT gene in those with artistic avocations and vocations compared to the general population. In the study by Ukkola-Vouti et al. previously referred to (2013), results implicated the GALM gene relevant for serotonin metabolism. These authors also in a previous study presented a substantial heritability estimate (0.84) for musical creativity (not included in the review) (Ukkola et al., 2009).

The neurophysiology of creativity

The second line of investigations into the biological aspects of creativity that has seen a surge recently is studies aimed at eliciting the *neurophysiological* underpinnings of creativity. The increase of studies in this area is in parallel with the development of new neuroimaging methodologies. More recently, researchers have tried to consolidate this seemingly disparate field, and attempted to review and suggest important goals for advancing the field (Arden et al., 2010; Dietrich and Kanso, 2010).

The split brain

There has been a considerable amount written about the right brain hemisphere and creativity (Runco, 2007a). Most of this has no bearing in empirical studies, but can rather be seen as irrelevant aspects of marketing commercialized training programmes in creativity. However, somewhat more balanced arguments of this view have also been held by prominent creativity scholars (Atchley et al., 1999), for example, Torrance (Torrance, 1982). Katz in his review of research on the left and right brain concluded that 'the simplistic argument [is] that the essential aspect of creativity resides in the right hemisphere. The claim that creativity is located "in" the right hemisphere (cf. Edwards 1979; Hendron 1989) should be dispelled with at once' (quoted in Runco, 2007a).

The idea of the right brain hemisphere being associated with creativity grew out of studies by Roger Sperry in the 1960s (1964). He investigated patients with epilepsy, who received surgery known as commissurotomy, in which the corpus callosum, a wide, flat bundle of neural fibres connecting the cerebral hemispheres, was destroyed resulting in a disconnecting of the two hemispheres. The purpose of the operation was to inhibit the spread or *generalization* of epileptic activity over the brain. However, the operation also made it possible to investigate the separate functions of the hemispheres, respectively. It was concluded that the right hemisphere specializes in parallel and global processes, whereas the left hemisphere mainly uses sequential and analytical processes (Katz, 1997; Sperry, 1964). In humans the left hemisphere is generally dominant. Sperry was not specifically investigating creative functioning. This was done more by, for example, Bogen and Bogen (1969), and Hoppe and Kyle (1990), who demonstrated that patients compared to controls exhibited a loss of emotional engagement, as well as an ability to understand symbolism (Runco, 2007a). They tended not to fantasize about, imagine, or interpret symbols. More recent research using, for example, fMRI have later provided some evidence that the right hemisphere is specifically implicated in creativity. For example, one study using fMRI saw activations in the right PFC in a creative story-generation task (Howard-Jones et al., 2005). However, on the whole studies do not support the premise that only one specific part of the brain is responsible for creativity, but instead that creativity is a global phenomenon of the brain.

Handedness and creativity

Handedness is sometimes investigated with the underlying assumption that this may aid as an indication of hemispheric dominance, in which nonright-handedness is conceived as a marker of disturbed brain lateralization (i.e., development of hemispheric dominance) (Preti and Vellante, 2007). There is some support for nonright-handedness being associated with creativity. Burke et al., for instance, investigating 12 left- and 12 right-handed college students found that left-handed individuals did slightly better on figural tests of divergent thinking but no differently in verbal divergent thinking (1989). There are also some reports of left-handed persons outnumbering the right-handed in creative and eminent samples (Peterson and Lansky, 1974, 1977). For example, one study reported that those left-handed were doubled (21 per cent) in students enrolled in architecture at the university level compared to what would be expected in the general population, and also saw proportionally more left-handed students than right-handed students graduating from the programme. Of 405 right-handed students, 251 (62 per cent) graduated; of 79 left-handed students, 58 (73.4 per cent) graduated. Similar findings have been made in mathematicians (Annett and Kilshaw, 1982), and musicians (Aggleton et al., 1994).

Studies have also reported nonright-handedness in psychopathologies (Annett and Kilshaw, 1982). Several studies report an excess of both mixed-handedness and left-handedness in schizophrenia (Dragovic and Hammond, 2005). In the general population, mixed-handedness is more often seen in people with high scores on measures of psychosis proneness, for example, schizotypy (Chapman and Chapman, 1987; Kim et al., 1992; Preti et al., 2007; Shaw et al., 2001).

One study specifically investigated the parallel findings of nonright-handedness in creativity and psychosis proneness (Preti et al., 2007). This study included 80 creative and 80 matched noncreative controls. Creative artists more often used their left hand than controls. They also scored higher on an inventory for psychosis proneness, although independently from their laterality score.

Structural neuroimaging

Studies investigating structural aspects of the brain in relation to creativity have been relatively few (Arden et al., 2010). Three studies from one research group used different methodologies to address this question; one used MRI to investigate anatomical structures (R.E. Jung, Segall et al., 2009), one used diffusion tensor imaging to investigate white matter in the brain (Jung, Grazioplene et al., 2010), and the third used magnetic resonance spectroscopy to investigate metabolites related to neuronal function (Jung, Gasparovic et al., 2009).

The first study of these studies (Jung, Segall et al., 2009), using volumetric MRI in a sample of 61 young adults found grey matter cortical thickness in a region in the lingual gyrus negatively associated with figural divergent thinking, but positively correlated with a different region in the right posterior cingulate. This study also obtained participants' scores on the CAQ (Carson et al., 2005), in which lower grey matter volume was associated with higher achieved creativity in the left lateral orbito-frontal region, but higher volume correlated with achieved creativity in the right angular gyrus. The authors suggested that 'a possible interpretation of our findings is that the generation of novel, original ideas is associated with less cortical thickness within frontal and (certain) posterior cortical regions, requiring higher functional activation to initiate cognitive control' (Jung, Segall et al., 2009), and stressed that results were not limited to *one lobe* of the brain, nor to one hemisphere, or suggesting that with regards to cortical thickness 'more is better', a notion otherwise characterizing cognitive neurosciences.

This conclusion was further stressed in the second study, which examined white matter integrity through diffusion tensor imaging (Jung, Grazioplene et al., 2010). This imaging method reveals the three dimensional diffusion of water providing information on neuronal axons (the nerve fibre conducting electrical impulses away from the neuron's cell body), since axons are coated with fatty myelin resulting in the diffusion of water to be greater along the axon length rather than perpendicular to it. The extent to which water diffuses in a principal direction is termed *fractional anisotropy*. If the fractional anisotropy value is high, it indicates that the white matter, which is partly derived from myelin, has a higher degree of structural integrity. Thus, axon bundles are roughly parallel and well insulated by myelin; low values of fractional anisotropy are indicative of lower structural coherence, resulting from compromised axonal integrity or less myelination. A positive correlation between IQ and the degree of fractional anisotropy has been reported previously (Schmithorst et al., 2005). However, Jung et al. (2010) found an inverse relationship between fractional anisotropy in the inferior frontal white matter and creativity, based on divergent thinking measurements assessed using the CAT. Areas involved were those linking the thalamus to prefrontal cortices. Interestingly, previous studies have also demonstrated lower fractional anisotropy in bipolar disorder and schizophrenia (McIntosh et al., 2008). The present study included tests for IQ and Big five personality traits (see Chapter 4). Fractional anisotropy in the right inferior frontal white matter was significantly inversely associated with *openness to experience*. Assessments of creativity were associated with both IQ and openness to experience. Further analyses suggested that findings of lower fractional anisotropy were due to lower levels of myelination rather than loss of axonal integrity. The findings in the two studies reviewed were corroborated by findings in the third study, which used magnetic resonance spectroscopy (Jung, Gasparovic et al., 2009). This study found an inversed correlation between the metabolite N-acetyl-aspartate (NAA) in right anterior grey matter and creativity. NAA is a marker of neuronal health and of relevance for myelin synthesis. Creativity in this study was similarly assessed as in the second study with CAT based on divergent thinking.

On the whole, the three studies using structural neuroimaging from the same research group suggest a left lateralized, fronto-subcortical, and *disinhibited* network of brain regions underlying creative cognition and achievement (Arden et al., 2010).

Functional neuroimaging

Functional neuroimaging refers to use of methods investigating dynamic processes in the brain. Studies using functional neuroimaging may be broadly categorized into a) Electroencephalography (EEG), b) fMRI c) PET and SPECT.

EEG studies

EEG uses a set of electrodes that are placed on the scalp in a standardized pattern. This allows for an investigation of voltage differences over the different electrodes over time, reflecting the direct communication of neurons. The main benefit of EEG is excellent temporal (millisecond) resolution; however, spatial resolution is lower. While the electric potential generated by a single neuron is far too weak to be picked up by EEG, the synchronous activity of many neurons having similar spatial orientation is strong enough to result in EEG activity. These oscillations thus represent synchronized activity over a network of neurons. Many of these oscillations have typical frequency ranges, spatial distributions and are linked to specific states of brain functioning (e.g., waking and the different sleep stages).

The majority of EEG studies conducted in conjunction to creativity show changes in the alpha band (range 8–12 Hz) (Arden et al., 2010). Increased power in this band is associated with attention and memory, while task performance is associated with alpha power suppression

(Klimesch, 1999). Arden et al. reviewed studies using EEG in relation to creativity in 2010 and found a total of 28 studies published between 1975 and 2009 (Arden et al., 2010). They concluded that these studies were provided by a limited number of research groups and that most used divergent thinking. However, many did not use standard assessment of divergent thinking, for example Guilford's utility test, but rather 'home-grown' measurements tapping into divergent thinking. Four studies used Guilford's test of divergent thinking, while four used the RAT. Other studies involved the use of such aspects of creativity as to mentally complete a drawing or imagining a dance improvisation (Bhattacharya and Petsche, 2002; Fink, Graif et al., 2009). While the diverse use of experimental paradigms clearly hampers the possibility to draw conclusions, some authors put forward that research in creativity also has been restrained by focusing too much on certain aspects, for example divergent thinking (Dietrich and Kanso, 2010). Thus there seems to be the need both for more studies using the same standardized instruments for specific aspects of creativity, while also allowing for the introduction of new experimental paradigms.

Three studies from three different research groups used the RAT, which established some convergent findings (Jung-Beeman et al., 2004; Martindale and Hines, 1975; Razumnikova, 2007). In summary, these studies all suggest a performance on the RAT to be linked to changes in alpha power (Arden et al., 2010). Martindale and Hines discussed these findings in comparison to findings with the Alternate uses test (i.e., Guildford's utility test), suggesting that the RAT was related with a tendency to vary amounts of alpha on different types of cognitive tasks, while creativity as measured by the Alternate uses test was found with a tendency to exhibit a high percentage of basal alpha overall. This would reflect that the Alternate uses test is primarily a measure of ideational fluency. As such, high scorers would consistently exhibit the broad, unfocused attention suggested by alpha abundance. The RAT, on the other hand, requiring both divergent and convergent (coming up with one right answer) thinking would see the need for both focusing and defocusing abilities (varying alpha power). These findings were further corroborated in other studies reviewed by Arden et al. (2010), as well as in a more recent study (Jauk et al., 2012). In all, however, findings in studies using EEG are heterogeneous, and it is difficult to draw any clear conclusions (Arden et al., 2010).

fMRI studies

The benefit of using fMRI is high spatial resolution. Whereas EEG has high temporal resolution, fMRI has higher spatial resolution, usually at about the level of a few millimetres (Arden et al., 2010). However, in the seven studies reviewed by Arden et al. (Asari et al., 2008; Fink, Grabner et al., 2009; Goel and Vartanian, 2005; Howard-Jones et al., 2005; Jung-Beeman et al., 2004; Kowatari et al., 2009; Mashal et al., 2007), none used the same experimental paradigm, and it is therefore difficult to draw any conclusions other than that different regions of the brain seem activated over the different paradigms. Regions implicated were, for example, those in frontal, temporal, and limbic lobes (Arden et al., 2010).

PET and SPECT studies

A few imaging studies have used PET and SPECT to investigate creativity. These methods reveal metabolic processes in the brain, and are based on the injection of radioactive ligands. While these investigations may provide information on receptor densities in the brain, most studies have used these methods to investigate cerebral blood flow, providing similar information as studies using fMRI (Arden et al., 2010; Bechtereva et al., 2004; Carlsson et al., 2000; Chavez-Eakle et al., 2007; Starchenko et al., 2003).

Thinking outside the box   An interesting study was performed by De Manzano et al., where PET was used to assess *DRD2 density* in relation to a measurement of divergent thinking (2010). Results demonstrated a negative correlation between divergent thinking and dopamine receptor-binding potential in the thalamus (Figure 5.1). Conceptualizing the thalamus as a central for information processing, the authors suggested that the result of this alteration would be a reduction in filtering of information flow (*noise*) and a subsequent excitation of cortical regions through decreased inhibition of prefrontal neurons. This would lead to a decrease in prefrontal signal-to-noise ratio, with prefrontal cortical regions more easily switching to a wider association range (an increase in divergent thinking). Conversely, this decreased signal-to-noise ratio should be disadvantageous in tasks that require high levels of selective attention, and lead to an increased risk of unwarranted signals from the thalamus overwhelming cortical neurotransmission resulting in cognitive disorganization and psychosis. In essence, the authors suggested that the decreased dopamine receptor-binding potential in the thalamus could reflect an increase of endogenous dopamine, resulting in thinking to be framed within a *less intact box*.

Dopamine metabolites in the cerebrospinal fluid   The idea that dopamine metabolism may be an important aspect of creative cognition has long

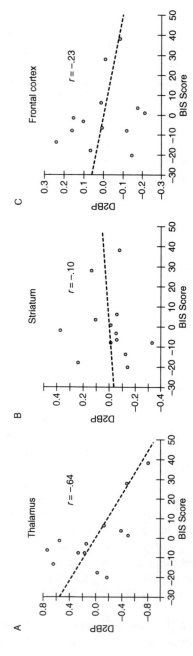

Figure 5.1 Correlations between divergent thinking (BIS score) scores and thalamic dopamine D2 binding potential.
Source: De Manzano et al., 2010.

been held (Flaherty, 2005). As was previously reviewed in this chapter, genes involved in dopamine metabolism have also been implicated in creativity (Murphy et al., 2013; Reuter et al., 2006; Runco et al., 2011). Flaherty suggested that the focused aspect of creative arousal, its high goal directedness, may be driven by mesolimbic dopaminergic activity (2005). In line with this, dopamine antagonists, generally used as antipsychotics, suppress free associations vital for creative cognition (Flaherty, 2005).

Dopamine activity is generally assessed by investigating homovanillic acid (HVA), a major dopamine metabolite (Amin et al., 1992). Three body fluids are accessible for quantifying HVA: cerebrospinal fluid (CSF), blood, and urine. In general CSF instead of blood or urine is preferred, since this provides the opportunity to estimate dopamine activity in the *brain*, without contribution of HVA from other tissues (Amin et al., 1992). However, the need to carry out lumbal puncture to accrue CSF generally makes CSF-HVA less available for research than routine blood or urine samples.

We recently assessed CSF-HVA in 73 healthy individuals and compared levels of CSF-HVA to the CAQ (Kyaga et al., 2014). This was the first study to directly measure a metabolite of dopamine in human cerebrospinal fluid in relation to assessed creativity. Surprisingly, rather than providing support for a positive correlation between dopamine activity and creativity, we found a significant inversed correlation between CSF-HVA and scores on the CAQ. Nevertheless, findings do not necessarily contradict previous suggestions of increased dopaminergic activity in the limbic system. The decrease in CSF-HVA might more accurately reflect a decrease of endogenous dopamine in prefrontal parts of the brain with sustained dopaminergic activity at, for example, the thalamus due to reduced density of D2 receptors (De Manzano et al., 2010). In line with this argument, in studies of monkeys, CSF-HVA reflects HVA in frontal cortical areas but not in other cortical areas (Elsworth et al., 1987). Further to the point, dopamine in the prefrontal cortex has been suggested as important for cognitive stability, while dopamine in sub-cortical regions may function to improve cognitive flexibility (Crofts et al., 2001; Van Schouwenburg et al., 2010).

Meta-analysis of neuroimaging in creativity

Neuroimaging experiments often fail to disclose neural substrates of cognitive processes. While one problem may be the question of how to operationalize the cognitive process investigated (e.g., creativity), another reason may be the use of limited sample sizes (Wang et al., 2010). Detecting a signal change of 0.5 per cent with 80 per cent power requires 25 or more participants (Wang et al., 2010), which is seldom seen in functional neuroimaging studies of creativity. Two recent reviews of neuroimaging in creativity highlight this fact (Arden et al., 2010; Dietrich and Kanso, 2010). One of these reviews (Dietrich and Kanso, 2010), is structured around three aspects of creativity; divergent thinking, artistic creativity, and insight, concluding that studies in the latter have the highest consistency.

We therefore conducted a meta-analysis (Figure 5.2) on 12 studies investigating insight using functional neuroimaging (Aziz-Zadeh et al.,

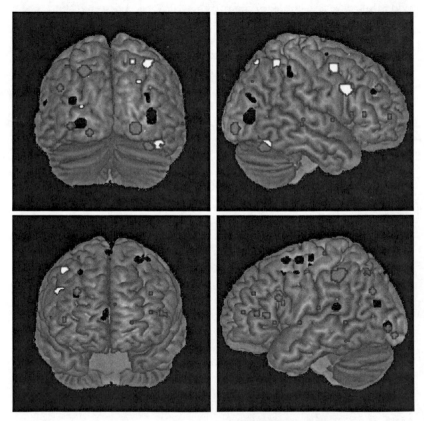

Figure 5.2   Meta-analysis of 12 studies investigating insight using functional neuroimaging.
Notes: Auditive experimental designs (black), visuo-spatial experimental designs (white) or semantic experimental designs (grey). Results did not support any common neural equivalent for insight.
Source: Kyaga and Liberg, 2010.

2009; Bechtereva et al., 2007; Bechtereva et al., 2004; Bengtsson et al., 2007; Carlsson et al., 2000; Fink, Grabner et al., 2009; Howard-Jones et al., 2005; Jung-Beeman et al., 2004; Kowatari et al., 2009; Limb and Braun, 2008; Mashal et al., 2007; Sieborger et al., 2007). We hypothesized that creativity, when defined as insight, would have a common neural correlate across creative domains. Studies were published 2004–9 and selected on the basis of searching the data bases PubMed, PsychINFO, and Web of Science, using the terms 'magnetic resonance imaging' *or* 'positron emission tomography' *and* 'creativeness'. Ten studies used fMRI, while two used PET. We classified experiments as auditive (music instrument improvisation), visuo-spatial (manipulation of spatial features) or semantic (manipulation of word use). We analysed activation with GingerALE 2.0 from BrainMap, Dallas TX, USA across all experiment types, but also for each type separately. Results did not support any common neural equivalent for insight (Kyaga and Liberg, 2010).

A more recent attempt by Gonen-Yaacovi et al. (2013), however, took a broader approach and included studies using functional neuroimaging to study different aspects of creativity. In all, 34 experiments with 622 healthy participants were included in the study. A total of 443 activation foci were included in the meta-analysis performed with GingerALE 2.2 from BrainMap, Dallas TX, USA. The authors performed both a global analysis, and also contrasted studies (in a subset of 29 experiments) using experimental designs based on combing information vs. self-generation of unusual responses (divergent thinking). The global analysis suggested that predominantly left-hemispheric regions were shared, including the caudal lateral PFC, the medial and lateral rostral PFC, and the inferior parietal and posterior temporal cortices. Contrasting studies based on combing information vs. self-generation of unusual responses, suggested that combination tasks activated more anterior areas of the lateral PFC than tasks including self-generation of unusual responses, though both types included caudal prefrontal areas (Figure 5.3). The lateral PFC was suggested to be structured along a rostro-caudal axis, with rostral regions involved in combining ideas and more posterior regions involved in creating novel ideas.

The prefrontal cortex

The PFC has received much interest from researchers in creativity (Gonen-Yaacovi et al., 2013; Runco, 2007a). It is considered responsible for higher mental functions, such as attention, working memory, and cognitive flexibility (Dietrich, 2004; Runco, 2007a). Interestingly, even direct manipulations of brain activity have been associated with

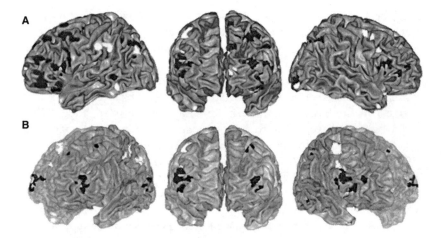

Figure 5.3   Meta-analysis of 34 experiments investigating creativity using functional neuroimaging.

Notes: (A) Combination task foci (black) and generation task foci (white). (B) Contrast studies of combination vs. generation tasks foci (black) and generation vs. combination task foci (white).

Source: Gonen-Yaacovi et al., 2013.

changes in creative and associated behaviours. By using rTMS Synder et al. created temporary 'lesions' of the fronto-temporal lobes in 11 healthy individuals (2003). Following this intervention research subjects created drawings considered by a committee as more life-like, flamboyant, and complex.

Nevertheless, the localizing of creativity to specific parts of the brain has been criticized (Dietrich, 2007). Arne Dietrich, a professor in cognitive neuroscience, suggests that research in creativity has been severely hampered by a sort of *monolithic* thinking, in which creative cognition and possibly creativity in general is considered to be just one thing. Dietrich stresses, for example, as has hopefully been made clear in this chapter, that 'creativity' is *not* in the right brain. This idea still prevailing in popular culture is suggested to have been the result of oversimplification by some scientists, further enhanced by ingenious journalists. More recent attempts to neuroanatomically pinpoint 'creativity' to the PFC is considered just another reincarnation of this fallacy. The underlying problem is the continual habit of treating creativity as a monolithic entity. Other examples of this bad habit, suggests Dietrich, is the idea that creativity equals divergent thinking, that creativity occurs only in a state of defocused attention or altered states of consciousness. The main aim for creativity research has to be to try to dissect the different aspects constituting the creative process. Of course, for creativity in general, other aspects, such as those relating to product and press (see Chapter 4) also need to be taken into consideration.

Dietrich provides a theoretical framework for a *cognitive neuroscience of creativity* (2004), in which the basic assumption is that neural circuits underlying noncreative information are essentially the same as those generating creative combinations of that information. This framework considers four basic types of creative cognition resulting from the combination of deliberate or spontaneous processing, and normative cognition or emotion; deliberate cognition, deliberate emotion, spontaneous cognition, and spontaneous emotion. These should not be seen as exclusive, but rather that creative behaviour in the end is the result of a mingling of these types.

In order to assess neuroanatomical correlates for these different types of creative processes, Dietrich acknowledges that the brain is structured according to a functional hierarchy, in which the PFC is placed as 'the zenithal higher order structure' (2004). Thus, the PFC is considered as essential for creativity, without necessarily suggesting that creativity resides within the PFC, but more to the point that aspects of creative cognition are contingent on the PFC. Essentially, once a creative idea has emerged it is subjected to a value assessment by the PFC, regardless of the type of creative process and neural circuit that generated the idea. This value assessment is essentially in parallel with the selection part of Campbell's and Simonton's *blind variation and selective retention* model of creativity discussed previously in Chapter 4 (Campbell, 1960; Simonton, 1999a).

Given that creative insight may develop both as the consequence of a deliberate problem-solving process, or spontaneously (Finke, 1996), Dietrich suggests that the former is the consequence of focused attention (2004), while the latter may result from defocused attention, such as daydreaming. The main difference between deliberate and spontaneous modes of processing is how unconscious novel information is represented in the *working memory*. A novel thought becomes a creative insight when it is represented in working memory. Information that is not represented in working memory is unconscious and thus inaccessible for reflection.

Deliberate searches for insights are initiated by circuits in the PFC and therefore are inclined to be rational, and conforming to internalized values and belief systems. The PFC can deliberately 'pull' task-relevant knowledge from long-term storage and temporarily represent it in the working memory. Once represented in the working memory, the PFC may use its capabilities to form new combinations (novel ideas). Thus, working memory capacity is critical for deliberate creativity, since it sets the limit on the number of possible ideational combinations. Given that an individual's cultural values and belief system are held within the PFC (Damasio, 1994), the search to retrieve knowledge is likely to be governed by the individual's already upheld world-view and previous experiences.

This practical rationality or 'common sense' has been difficult to conceptualize (Owen et al., 2007). In general it is suggested to denote a form of knowing that offers the contextual assumptions about the world forming the basis of shared human existence. Such knowledge is generally taken for granted and used every day. Interestingly, patients with schizophrenia have been argued to be impaired in common sense, but also found to be less restrained by it in making correct logical deductions, when in contrast to common sense truth (Owen et al., 2007).

Patients with schizophrenia and those at risk of developing schizophrenia have consistently demonstrated structural abnormalities in the PFC. These have been present in both dorsolateral PFC (DLPFC), as well as in medial PFC (MPFC) and the anterior cingulate cortex (ACC) (Jung, Jang et al., 2010). Alterations in common sense could reflect the latter two brain regions (MPFC and ACC), which in a recent review was suggested to be implicated in self-related processing (Nelson et al., 2009). Thus, MPFC and ACC may reflect the selectional aspect of Campbell's and Simonton's *blind variation and selective retention* model of creativity discussed in Chapter 4 (Campbell, 1960; Simonton, 1999a), while DLPFC is accountable for set shifting, i.e., cognitive flexibility. The latter is evident by perseveration or the inability to shift between modes of thinking, being the most reliable deficit associated with damage to the DLPFC (Boone, 1998; Dietrich, 2004).

However, this perseveration does not necessary suggest cognitive stability, but rather reflects the loss of inhibitory control over maladaptive emotional and cognitive behaviours. Flexible, adaptive behaviour requires cognitive *control*; the capacity to manage one's own thoughts and actions in accord with internally represented goals (Cieslik et al., 2013). DLPFC has consistently been associated with cognitive control. In parallel, previously discussed alpha waves in prefrontal EEG in creativity are conceived to indicate top-down control actively inhibiting task-irrelevant activity such as irrelevant sensory processing or the retrieval of interfering information (Fink and Benedek, 2012; Klimesch, 2012). Thus, the DLPFC may be regarded as responsible for the *retention* part of Campbell's and Simonton's *blind variation and selective retention* model of creativity (Campbell, 1960; Simonton, 1999a).

Spontaneous insights instead happen when the attentional system does not actively choose the content of consciousness, which allows for unfiltered *random* unconscious thoughts to be represented in working memory (Dietrich, 2004). Thus, ideas that are not guided by common sense and societal norms, or theoretical rationality, suddenly become represented in working memory. There is an *element of chance* in which ideas will be represented. Dietrich suggests that an evident example of this is in REM sleep, which is marked by prefrontal inactivity, resulting in dreams in which self-reflection is absent, time is distorted, volitional control is minor, and few suggestions of active decision making or focused attention are present. But where do the ideational combinations, that is, the blind variation in the *blind variation and selective retention* model of creativity emancipate? Dietrich suggests, that by drawing from already existing knowledge in cognitive neuroscience, it can be concluded that the same neural circuits that process specific information to yield noncreative ideas must be the same neural circuits that are responsible for the generation of creative combinations of that information (Dietrich, 2004, 2007). The information resulting in the *blind variation* of novel ideas must originate in the very neural circuits that are keeping the specific information. This is granted merely on the appreciation of the brain as a nonlinear information processor; novelty is intrinsic in such a complex system (Dietrich, 2007).

Summary

Most studies investigating putative genetic underpinnings for creativity affirm a genetic component in creativity. However, results are hampered by different methods to measure creativity and also by stemming from comparable small cohorts. More recently, attempts to specifically invest candidate genes implicated in creativity have been directed at those related to monoaminergic systems, for example the dopamine system, and neuronal development. As yet, none of these studies have used a genome-wide approach on a large scale. This means that findings need to be considered with caution and subjected to replication before any clear conclusions can be drawn, though genes implicated in dopamine metabolism may be considered partly replicated. In order for the field to progress, there appears to be a need to consolidate present findings and possibly to coordinate attempts for large-scale studies using more systematic approaches to molecular genetics. Considering that creativity is a complex trait, it seems highly unlikely that any one gene will contribute to but a small fraction of the variance of creativity.

In parallel with the increase of studies investigating the genetical underpinnings of creativity, recent advances in neuroimaging have also led to new approaches in forming a cognitive neuroscience of creativity. Several attempts have been made to consolidate the field (Arden et al., 2010; Dietrich and Kanso, 2010; Fink and Benedek, 2012; Gonen-Yaacovi et al., 2013). While these have been able to discard simplified ideas of 'creativity' residing in the right hemisphere, many studies have instead implicated the PFC in creative cognition. This has led some researcher to call for a new approach in research on creative cognition that does not spring from the perspective of creativity being inherently different from other types of cognition, but rather resulting from the same neural circuits responsible for noncreative cognition. Given this view, it is suggested that the different constituents of creative cognition needs to be differentiated and more clearly defined. Without resorting to localizing 'creativity' in the PFC, it is suggested that the PFC may function as a final pathway holding functions parallel to selection and retention in Campbell's and Simonton's *blind variation and selective retention* model of creativity (Campbell, 1960; Simonton, 1999a), while the blind variation of novel ideas are born in the very neural circuits holding the specific knowledge (Dietrich, 2007).

6
Contemporary Studies on Creativity and Psychopathology

Introduction

The mad genius link remains one of the most heated debates in contemporary research on creativity (Silvia and Kaufman, 2010). Authors hold completely opposing positions; some contending that psychopathology have nothing to do with creativity (Rothenberg, 1995; Sawyer, 2012b; Schlesinger, 2009, 2012), while others assert the two to be profoundly associated (Andreasen, 2008; Jamison, 1996; Ludwig, 1995). Discussions on the topic are often collared by strong emotions and less often founded on empirical research (Silvia and Kaufman, 2010). The current chapter therefore aims to present a complete overview of original contemporary research conducted on the question of creativity and psychopathology, while also discussing the results of these studies in relation to some of the major criticism that has been evoked by these studies.

Literature review

A total of 98 original studies, make up the core of this review (Kyaga, 2014). Most studies reviewed are aimed at psychotic disorders, such as schizophrenia or bipolar disorder, or subsyndromal psychotic features, for example schizotypy. Concurrent with explorations on subsyndromal symptoms, a number of studies also include non-diagnosed relatives of patients. These studies are also of relevance for suggestions of a genetic mechanism underlying the putative association between creativity and psychopathology.

Search strategy

The search strategy for the review was based on the following criteria: all articles, letters, meeting abstracts or book chapters published in English attained through the MESH-terms 'creativity' *and* 'mental disorder' in the databases MEDLINE and Web of Science. The search yielded a total number of 690 and 140 hits, respectively, which after examining the titles and abstracts were pruned to include exclusively original studies. This resulted in a total of 98 original studies published until December 2013. One study was published in 1959, whereas all other studies were published after 1970. Articles are presented according to five broad categories: a) studies investigating psychotic and mood disorders (Table 6.1), b) studies primarily investigating neurodevelopmental disorders (Table 6.2), c) studies primarily investigating substance use/abuse disorders (Table 6.3), d) studies primarily investigating neurological disorders (Table 6.4), and e) studies investigating other mental disorders (Table 6.5).

Psychotic and mood disorders

The major part of studies reviewed is directed at psychotic disorders, such as schizophrenia and bipolar disorder. One important reason for this is most likely that schizophrenia and bipolar disorder can be characterized as the prototypical severe psychiatric illnesses, which have defined psychiatry since the late nineteenth century (Shorter, 1997). There has also been an animated discussion whether schizophrenia or rather bipolar disorder is linked to creativity. An example of this difference of opinions can be found in the *Journal of Creativity Research*, in which Louis A. Sass criticized the conclusions by Kay Redfield Jamison and others, who argued for a link between bipolar disorder and creativity (2000b). Sass attacked Jamison for an overly romantic view of creativity, not corresponding to how creativity was expressed in a more modernist and postmodern time. Jamison replied that she in no way questioned that creativity to a certain extent is time and culture bound, or the possibility of a link between schizophrenia and creativity (2000). However, she said that at the time there was empirical support for an association between bipolar disorder and creativity, while this was not present for schizophrenia and creativity. In the years following this dispute, additional studies have been performed, and they have in several cases suggested support for a link between bipolar disorder and creativity, without correspondingly providing similar support for an association between schizophrenia disorder and creativity. However, quite a few studies have suggested a connection between *subsyndromal* psychotic symptoms (e.g., schizotypy) and creativity. Schizotypal traits can be broadly categorized into three groups: positive schizotypy (e.g., unusual cognitive and perceptual experiences, tendency to magical ideation,

Table 6.1 Summary of studies investigating psychotic and affective disorders

Reference	Study sample	Assessment of mental disorder	Definition of creativity	Findings
(Herbert, 1959)	60 patients admitted to The New York Hospital Westchester Division 1928 to 1955.	Personality disorders, addiction, psychoneuroses, schizophrenia, paranoid, manic-depressive, melancholia, organic mental reactions.	Artistic occupation.	• Increase in personality disorders—diagnosed as 'psychopathic personality'.
(Karlsson, 1970)	486 relatives of psychotic persons born 1881-1910, identified from the records of the Kleppur Mental Hospital in Reykjavik, Iceland. Relatives were born 1851-1940. Three kindreds and their branches were specifically investigated.	Schizophrenia: n = 362, manic depressive: n = 124.	Listed in the Who's Who.	• First-degree and second-degree relatives of patients more often listed in Who's Who compared to the general population. • Same branches are high in both psychosis and listings in Who's Who.
(Andreasen and Powers, 1975)	15 creative writer, manic (n = 16) and schizophrenic (n = 15) patients.	Consecutive series of maniacs and schizophrenics admitted to the University of Iowa Psychiatric Inpatient Service.	Writers from the University of Iowa Writers' Workshop.	• Writers and maniacs showed more behavioural and conceptual over-inclusion, but writers showed substantially more richness and the manics more idiosyncratic thinking. • Schizophrenics tended to be under-inclusive rather than over-inclusive and showed less richness and bizarreness than the writers and maniacs.

(continued)

Table 6.1 Continued

(Dykes and Mcghie, 1976)	300 university students, 24 acute non-paranoid schizophrenic patients. From the 300 students the 24 highest scoring and the 24 lowest scoring subjects were extracted from the total group to represent our two extreme creativity groups.	Patients given a diagnosis of schizophrenia (made independently by two psychiatrists) and with an above-average verbal IQ.	Lovibond Object Sorting Test (divergent thinking), Chapman Card Sorting Test (convergent thinking), Dichotic Shadowing Task (assessing the degree to which each subject assimilates the information in both the relevant and irrelevant and the effect of the intrusion of irrelevant material on performance).	• Similarities in attentional strategies in creative and schizophrenic individuals, both groups appeared to sample a wider range of environmental input. • This widening of attention appeared to be involuntary in the schizophrenic, resulting in a deleterious effect on performance.
(al-Issa, 1976)	50 schizophrenics.	Patients were randomly selected from a hospital population and rated with the Activity-Withdrawal scale constructed by Venables and Epstein Inclusion Test.	10 tests for creative abilities as described by Guilford.	• Level of education and vocabulary are positively related to creativity scores, over-inclusion, activity-withdrawal, and age tend to show the opposite trend.
(Kidner, 1976)	68 volunteers of British nationality.	Eysenck Psychoticism and Neuroticism scales, Raven's Advanced Progressive Matrices test and the Mill Hill Vocabulary test served as intelligence indices. Acceptance of Culture scale, was used as an index of socialization.	Wallach and Kogan's Object Uses, Similarities, and Pattern Meanings tests, scored for both fluency and originality.	• Creativity correlated positively with Eysenck's Psychoticism scale, and negatively with the Acceptance of Culture scale.
(Schou, 1979)	24 manic-depressive artists with lithium treatment were interviewed about their creative power during the treatment.	Manic-depressive illness, bipolar or unipolar, in whom prophylactic lithium treatment had been successful.	Artistic occupation.	• 12 artists reported increased artistic productivity, 6 unaltered productivity, and 6 lowered productivity.

(Kauffman et al., 1979)	6 most competent children to 30 mothers with schizophrenia, bipolar or unipolar affective psychosis compared to 6 most competent children of mothers without any psychiatric disorder.	Anthony's six point scale. Ratings of maternal and paternal psychosocial functioning were based on the Strauss-Carpenter structured interview.		• The children from healthy families were not as creative as those in the high competence group of mothers with psychiatric disorders.
(Phillips, 1982)	8 patients with bipolar disorder receiving lithium treatment.	In clinical care by the author.	2 patients were artists.	• Impression that lithium maintenance treatment does not, in most instances, exert a negative influence on creativity.
(Tucker et al., 1982)	74 final year students in high school.	Allusive (loose) thinking in Rapaport-Lovibond Object Sorting Test (OST).	Wallach and Kogan test, peer-rated creativity, assessment of creative activities, Holland Vocational Preference Inventory (VPI) Artistic Scale, Mill Hill Vocabulary Scale.	• When the effect of intelligence was accounted for, there was a relationship between peer-rated creativity and OST scores.
(Tucker et al., 1982)	Sydney's art galleries were asked to list 10 artists in Sydney whom they considered to be most creative. 12 artists accepted to participate.	Allusive (loose) thinking in Rapaport-Lovibond Object Sorting Test (OST).	The Kent-Rosanoff Word Association Test, Mill Hill Vocabulary Scale, Wallach and Kogan Creativity Test.	• Compared with administrators, visual artists had higher scores on OST.

(continued)

Table 6.1 Continued

(Rothenberg, 1983)	12 Nobel laureates (scientists), 18 hospitalized patients, and 113 college students.	Students were divided into high (63) and low (50) creative groups on the basis of a quantitative assessment of their creative achievements in the arts and sciences. Each subject responded to 99 stimulus words. Word association responses were classified as opposite, primary, and other.	• Number of responses and speed of responses were sharply different within each creative group, and the group with proved creativity, the Nobel laureates, gave the highest number of opposite responses at the fastest rate of all groups. • The patient group did not show a tendency to rapid opposite responding.
(Karlsson, 1984)	8007 relatives of psychotic persons born 1881-1910 were compared to the general population. The relatives were born 1851-1940.	Graduates of the Reykjavik Gymnasium college, authors of published books or listed in the Who's Who.	• The relatives were overrepresented as graduates (2.5% vs 2.0%), authors (2.0% vs 1.3%), and in Who's Who (4.2% vs 3.4%).
(Kline and Cooper, 1986)	Healthy students (n = 173; 96 females and 77 males).	Eysenck Personality Questionnaire. Scales from the Comprehensive Ability Battery (Flexibility of Closure, Spontaneous Flexibility, Ideational Fluency, Word Fluency, Originality).	• Only Word Fluency in males demonstrated a significant association.
(Shaw et al., 1986)	DSM-III criteria: 20 patients who completed the protocol had bipolar disorder, 1 recurrent depressive disorder, 1 bipolar disorder (mixed). The patients had been receiving lithium therapy for a mean period of 9.4 years at mean lithium level of 0.80 mmol/liter.	22 euthymic patients. The first, fourth and fifth week was with active lithium, whereas week two and three were with placebo. Palermo and Jenkins' Word Association Norms. Associative idiosyncrasy or quality was measured by comparing the subject's associations to those norms. Words included by the patient that were not on the list were judged to be idiosyncratic.	• Lithium discontinuation produced a significant increase in associational productivity and a demonstrable increase in associative idiosyncrasy. Restoration of lithium dose significantly reversed both effects.

(Andreasen, 1987)	Rates of mental illness were examined in 30 creative writers (3 females, 27 males), 30 matched control subjects, and the first-degree relatives of both groups.	Structured interview designed by the. The probands were diagnosed according to the Research Diagnostic Criteria (RDC), and diagnoses of first-degree relatives were made according to the Family History Research Diagnostic Criteria.	The creative writers were drawn from a sample at the University of Iowa Writers' Workshop. A subset of 15 writers and control subjects: Raven Progressive Matrices and the WAIS.	• 80% of the writers had had an episode of affective illness, compared with 30% of the control subjects. • 43% of the writers had had bipolar illness, compared with 10% of the controls. • Writers had higher rates of alcoholism (30%, compared with 7% in the controls).
(Richards et al., 1988)	17 manic-depressives, 16 cyclothymes, and 11 healthy first-degree relatives to patients were compared with 33 controls with no personal or family history of major affective disorder, cyclothymia, or schizophrenia; 15 controls were healthy and 18 carried another diagnosis.	DSM-III with primary or secondary diagnosis of manic-depressive illness. Controls having neither personal nor a family history of major affective disorder or cyclothymia, bipolar disorder, or schizophrenia or suicide.	Lifetime Creativity Scales.	• Creativity significantly higher among the combined index subjects (manic-depressive, cyclothymes, and normal relatives) than among controls. • No significant difference between normal and ill controls. • Suggestively higher creativity among normal index relatives than among manic-depressives (p < .10).
(Schuldberg et al., 1988)	College students, who rated high on scales measuring schizotypy (n = 52; 23 females, 29 males) were compared with controls (n = 65; 32 females, 33 males).	The perceptual aberration scale, Magical ideation scale, Physical anhedonia scale, an infrequency scale. Subjects scoring > 2 SD on Perceptual aberration or Magical ideation. Controls scored max ½ SDs above the mean.	The quick word test, Alternate uses test, BWAS, ACL, and How do you think.	• Association between schizotypal positive symptoms and the creativity tests. • This association was due to two tests: BWAS and How do you think.

(continued)

Table 6.1 Continued

(Jamison, 1989)	Poets, playwrights, novelists, biographers and artists (n = 47).	Open-ended and scaled questions about history and type of treatment. Specific diagnostic criteria were not used.	• 38% of the total sample had been treated for an affective illness. • The playwrights had the highest total rate of treatment for affective illness (63%). • Only poets (16.7%) were treated for bipolar illness with hospitalization, lithium, ECT, etc.
(Ludwig, 1992)	1005 individuals.	Those whose biographies were reviewed in the *New York Times Book Review* 1960-1990. Creative Achievement Scale (CAS).	• Those in creative arts had higher rates of alcoholism, drug abuse, depression, mania, somatic problems, anxiety, psychoses, and adjustment disorders. • Theatrical professions demonstrated comparably high rates of alcohol and drug abuse, mania, anxiety disorders, and suicide attempts. • Writers of fiction and poets shared alcohol and drug abuse, depression, and suicide attempts. • Artists had comparably high rates of alcohol abuse, depression, anxiety, and adjustment problems. • Musical composers had especially heightened rates of alcohol abuse and depression.

(Post, 1994)	Family background, physical health, personality, psychosexuality, and mental health of 291 famous men in science, thought, politics, and art were investigated.	Based on biographies, extracted data were transformed into diagnoses in accordance with DSM-III-R criteria, when appropriate.	Subjects chosen were those judged to have achieved lasting international fame for their innovations in a variety of fields. Only biographies, which had been published sometime after the subjects' deaths were used.	<ul><li>In general, these men were emotionally warm, with a gift for friendship and sociability.</li><li>Most had unusual personality characteristics and severe personality deviations were unduly frequent only in the case of visual artists (20%) and writers (25%).</li><li>Functional psychoses were entirely restricted to the affective varieties.</li><li>Among other disorders, only depressive conditions and alcoholism, were more prevalent and strikingly so in writers (72% resp. 14%).</li></ul>
(Ludwig, 1994)	Questionnaire and interview data were obtained on 59 female writers and 59 members of a matched comparison group.	A series of standard inventories (e.g., Sensation-Seeking Scale, Rotter I-E Scale, Personal Reaction Inventory, Maudsley Personality Inventory, and Ways of Coping Checklist). Questionnaire for DSM-III-R criteria, in subjects and their biological parents and siblings.	Modified version Lifetime Creativity Scales and semi-structured Interviews.	<ul><li>Writers were more likely to suffer from depression, bipolar disorder, drug abuse, panic attacks, generalized anxiety, eating disorders, and nonspecific emotional disorders.</li><li>The parents (in particular, the mothers) of the female writers were more likely to suffer from some sort of mental illness than those of the comparison group.</li><li>Higher percentages of writers than members of the comparison group reported experiencing sexual and physical abuse before the age of 13.</li></ul>

(continued)

Table 6.1 Continued

			• Writers were more likely than comparison subjects to identify their sexual orientations as homosexual or bisexual. • Writers displayed higher overall scores on the Life time Creativity Scales than the comparison group. • Marked creative activity in mothers, fathers, or any siblings resulted in an increased likelihood for a writer as a first-degree relative.
(Sitton and Hughes, 1995)	14 men and 44 women in undergraduate psychology classes and from a local writers' organization (6 women, 2 men).	Beck depression inventory and a 16-item questionnaire dealing with atypical symptoms of depression, including seasonal variation in mood and productivity.	• Fall was designated as the most productive season significantly more frequently than other seasons. • Failure to find a correlation between current depressive state and creativity.
(Sitton and Hughes, 1995)	College students (33 men and 67 women).	–	RAT.
		Brief questionnaire regarding perceptions of their creative processes, specifying any seasonal or daily variations in creativity. Thematic Apperception Test. Creativity of the stories was evaluated by judges.	• No seasonal differences in the ratings of the stories. • Those who rated fall as their most creative season wrote stories rated as more creative than those who preferred spring regardless of the season in which they wrote.

(Post, 1996)	~100 well-known American and British prose and play writers were included. Living poets and those who had died before the 1840s were excluded.	Anthologies of English (Gardner, 1972) and American (Ellmann, 1976) verse supplied the names of poets selected by experts. Based on biographies, extracted data were transformed into diagnoses in accordance with DSM-III-R criteria, when appropriate.	• Prevalence of dysfunctional personality traits (30%) was much higher than the 13% prevalence reported by Tyrer et al (1991) in a general population. • Psychopathology within the affective spectrum was found in 80.0% of poets, 80.5% of novelists/ poets, and in 87.5% of playwrights. Eight writers committed suicide, and this 8% rate exceeded the 1980 rates of 0.73–0.84% for England and Wales as well as the 1.89–2.17 for Austria (World Health Organization, 1983). • Alcoholism was at its lowest in poets (31%) and highest in playwrights (54%). • The prevalence of bi- and homosexuality exceeded the population norm of 11.9% (Johnson et al, 1992) only in playwrights with 29%.
(Karlsson, 1999)	Relatives of 1377 index cases with a psychotic diagnosis.	The 6 best mathematics performers aged 20 each year during a 30-year period based on scores assigned in the mathematics examination at the Reykjavik College. Admitted to a mental hospital.	• A 3% rate of hospitalization among the top mathematicians and their siblings. • There were 18 instances of psychosis instead of expected 5.

(continued)

Table 6.1 Continued

(Ghadirian et al., 2000)	20 patients with bipolar disorder and 24 patients suffering from other psychopathologies (schizophrenia, depression, and personality disorder) (23 females and 21 males).	Clinical diagnosis was established by a psychiatrist on the basis of DSM-III diagnostic criteria. All patients were assessed as: recovered, mildly ill, moderately ill, or severely ill.	A battery of tests measuring creativity in nonverbal, visual–motor, perceptual, and verbal subtests.	• There was no significant difference in creativity between the two groups with bipolar disorder and other psychopathologies, respectively. • The group of patients identified as severely ill showed significantly lower levels of creativity, than the three other groups.
(Kinney et al., 2000)	36 adult adoptees of biological parents with schizophrenia, and 36 control adoptees with no biological family history of psychiatric hospitalization.	DSM-III, based on structured interview.	Lifetime Creativity Scales	• Non-schizophrenics with either schizotypal or schizoid personality disorder or multiple schizotypal signs had significantly higher creativity than other participants.
(Weinstein and Graves, 2002)	60 undergraduates. 21 men (3 non-right-handed) and 39 women (4 were non-right-handed).	Edinburgh Handedness Inventory, Magical Ideation, Perceptual Aberration, Revised Social Anhedonia, 13 infrequency items. Stimuli for the lexical decision task were 15 four-letter English words and 45 four-letter nonsense words. The dichotic listening task (DLT) stimuli were six natural voice, consonant–vowel (CV) nonsense syllables produced.	Shortened version of the RAT, Thurstone Written Fluency Test.	• Creativity and schizotypy (per-mag) are correlated. • Creativity and schizotypy (per-mag) are partly related to a response criterion favouring right hemisphere. • Dichotic listening results revealed a strong association of better right hemisphere (left ear) localization ability and creativity.

Study	Sample	Measures		Results
(Papworth and James, 2003)	104 undergraduate students (N = 36 art and 68 science)	Depression Adjective Check List, Cognitive Distortion Questionnaire.	TTCT, Means-Ends Problem Solving Procedure.	• Art students were found to be more creative, experienced lower mood, and displayed greater degrees of distortion and bias in their appraisals.
(Ramey and Weisberg, 2004)	Emily Dickinson's creative productivity over the course of her career was examined to test the hypothesis that mood disorder affects creative thinking.	–	Franklin's (1998) collection of Dickinson's poetry was used to determine the date of each of Dickinson's poems. 19 anthologies of poetry and tabulated the number of Dickinson's poems that were present in each to investigate quality.	• During the years with Seasonal affective disorder, a significant increase was found in quality of poems produced during autumn + winter. This relationship did not hold for the hypomanic years.
(Nowakowska et al., 2005)	49 bipolar patients (BP), 25 with major depressive disorder (MDD), 32 creative controls (CC), and 47 healthy controls (HC) completed self-report temperament/personality measures.	TEMPS-A, NEO-PI-R, and the Temperament and Character Inventory (TCI). Structured Clinical Interview (SCID) for DSM-IV Diagnosis was conducted by a psychiatrist or experienced research coordinator to determine presence or absence of psychiatric disorders, and confirm euthymic mood state.	CC's were volunteers with no current psychiatric or substance abuse problems, recruited from graduate programs in creative writing, fine arts, and product design at Stanford University.	• Euthymic BP, MDD, and CC, compared to HC, had significantly increased cyclothymia, dysthymia and irritability scores on TEMPS-A; increased neuroticism and decreased conscientiousness on NEO-PI-R; and increased harm avoidance and novelty seeking as well as decreased self-directedness on TCI. • TEMPS-A cyclothymia scores were significantly higher in BP than in MDD. • NEO-PI-R openness was increased in BP and CC, compared to HC, and in CC compared to MDD. • TCI self-transcendence scores in BP were significantly higher than in MDD, CC, and HC.

(continued)

Table 6.1 Continued

Study	Sample	Measures	Findings
(Schuldberg, 2005)	625 undergraduate students.	Eysenck Personality Questionnaire, Wisconsin scales of hypothetical Psychosis-proneness and Hypomanic traits, the Golden and Meehl Schizoid taxon scale.	Alternate uses, Revised Art Scale, How Do You Think, Gough's Adjective Checklist creativity scale, RAT.	• The Psychoticism scores were correlated (.30) with Hypomanic traits, (.25) with Perceptual Aberration, and (.20) with the How Do You Think. • Psychoticism scores were negatively related to Remote Associates Test. Extraversion scores were correlated (.45) with How Do You Think, and (.37) with Adjective Checklist.
(Simeonova et al., 2005)	40 adults with bipolar disorder (BD), 20 bipolar offspring with BD, 20 bipolar offspring with ADHD, and 18 healthy control parents and their 18 healthy control children.	Structured Clinical Interview for DSM-IV Axis I Disorders (SCID), Family History-Research Diagnostic Criteria (FH-RDC), WASH-U-KSADS, K-SADS-PL, YMRS, CDRS-R. All evaluations were conducted by either a child and adolescent psychiatrist or a master level research assistant.	BWAS.	• Adults with BD compared to controls scored (120%) higher on the BWAS Dislike subscale, and non-significantly (32%) higher on the BWAS Total scale. • Mean BWAS Dislike subscale scores were higher in offspring with BD (107% higher) and offspring with ADHD (91% higher) than in healthy control children. • In the bipolar offspring with BD, BWAS Total scores were negatively correlated with duration of illness.
(Folley and Park, 2005)	17 outpatient schizophrenic (SZ) subjects. 17 healthy control (CO) and 17 schizotypal (SCT). 10 SZ, 10 SCT and 10 CO participated in near-infrared optical spectroscopy (NIRS) part of the study.	DSM-IV. Brief Psychiatric Rating Scale (BPRS), Scales for the Assessment of Positive (SAPS) and Negative (SANS) Symptoms, Schizotypal Personality Questionnaire (SPQ), Wechsler Abbreviated Scales of Intelligence, Edinburgh Handedness Inventory. NIRS was performed using a 24-channel spectrometer.	RAT and a novel divergent thinking task (DT) based on earlier models of creativity. Fluency was measured using verbal (FAS) category, and design (Five Point Test) fluency tasks.	• CO gave more correct responses than schizophrenics on the RAT. • SCT had enhanced DT ability compared with SZ and CO, who showed similar performance overall. • NIRS data showed that DT was associated with bilateral prefrontal cortex (PFC) activation, but the right PFC particularly contributed to the enhanced creative thinking in SCT compared with the other two groups.

Study	Sample	Measures	Findings
(Nettle and Clegg, 2006)	425 British adults (156 male, 269 female).	O-LIFE schizotypy inventory and a section on psychiatric history and information on mating success ('Since you were 18, how much of the time have you been in a steady relationship?' and 'Since you were 18, how many different partners have you?').	Participants indicated their degree of creative activity in poetry or visual art. Participants rated themselves as not producing poetry or art (241 participants), being a hobby producer (57), a serious producer (60) or a professional producer (67) in either domain.	• Positive relationships between *unusual experiences* and mating success, and *impulsive non-conformity* and mating success. • In *unusual experiences*, this relationship was mediated by creative activity. • In *impulsive non-conformity*, this relationship was not mediated by creative activity. • *Introvertive anhedonia* decreased creative activity, and also had a direct negative effect on mating success.
(Nettle, 2006)	501 individuals (309 healthy, 168 affective disorder, 13 schizophrenia, 11 bipolar disorder).	Psychopathology was rated from answers to detailed questions about symptoms and treatment. O-LIFE schizotypy.	Poets, visual artists, mathematicians.	• Poets and artists had levels of *unusual experiences* that were higher than controls, and as high as schizophrenia patients. However, they were relatively low on the dimension of *introvertive anhedonia*. • Mathematicians were lower than controls on *unusual experiences*.

(continued)

Table 6.1 Continued

(Burch et al, 2006)	107 undergraduate and postgraduate students.	O-LIFE, NEO-FFI, Wechsler abbreviated scale of intelligence	53 students were recruited from the Department of Visual Arts. Remaining 54 participants were all non-artists. Creative personality scale, Instances and Uses tests of divergent thinking.	• Largest difference between the visual artists and non-artists occurred on *unusual experience* scores of the O-LIFE. • Visual artists scored higher than non-artists on cognitive disorganization, impulsive nonconformity, neuroticism, openness and divergent thinking (uniqueness), while non-artists scored higher on agreeableness. • Males generally scored higher on both divergent thinking uniqueness and totals scores, IQ and impulsive nonconformity scores.
(Abraham et al., 2007)	28 patients with schizophrenia (SZ) and 18 healthy controls.	Schedules for assessment of positive and negative symptoms (SAPS and SANS) of the Comprehensive Assessment of Symptoms and History (CASH). Digit backward span, Hayling sentence completion test, Brixton spatial anticipation test, Stroop Neuropsychological Screening Test.	Ward animal task, Creative imagery, Constraints of examples, Alternate uses, Convergent (insight and incremental) problem solving.	• In executive function measures, except Hayling task on which no significant difference in performance was found between the groups, SZ had poorer performance than the control group on all the other executive tasks. • In creative cognition measures, SZ were poorer in performance on insight problem, incremental problem, imagery measure, alternate uses uniqueness, and the alternate uses fluency.

| (Santosa et al., 2007) | 49 patients with bipolar disorder (BP), 25 Major depressive disorder (MDD), 32 creative controls (CC), and 47 healthy controls (HC) (all euthymic). | Medical and psychiatric history and Structured Clinical Interview for DSM-IV Diagnosis (SCID) by a psychiatrist or experienced research coordinator. Psychiatrist utilizing a semi-structured interview confirmed that subjects were euthymic. | BWAS, the Adjective Check List Creative Personality Scale, and the TTCT – Figural (TTCT-F) and Verbal versions. | • BP and CC (but not MDD) compared to HC scored significantly higher on BWAS-Total and BWAS-Dislike, but not on BWAS-Like.
• CC compared to MDD scored significantly higher on TTCT-F. |
| (Strong et al., 2007) | 49 patients with bipolar disorder (BP), 25 Major depressive disorder (MDD), 32 creative controls (CC), and 47 healthy controls (HC) (all euthymic). | Medical and psychiatric history and Structured Clinical Interview for DSM-IV Diagnosis (SCID) by a psychiatrist or experienced research coordinator. Psychiatrist utilizing a semi-structured interview confirmed that subjects were euthymic. Revised NEO Personality Inventory (NEO-PI-R), the TEMPS-A, and the Temperament and Character Inventory (TCI). | BWAS, the Adjective Check List Creative Personality Scale, and the TTCT – Figural (TTCT-F) and Verbal versions. | • Neuroticism/Cyclothymia/ Dysthymia Factor, comprised mostly of NEO-PI-R-Neuroticism and TEMPS-A-Cyclothymia and TEMPS-A-Dysthymia, was related to BWAS-Total scores and BWAS-Dislike subscale scores.
• An Openness Factor, comprised mostly of NEO-PI-R-Openness, was related to BWAS-Like subscale scores, and to ACL-CPS scores. |

(continued)

Table 6.1 Continued

| (Miller and Tal, 2007) | 225 University of New Mexico students. | Schizotypy (SPQ), NEO–FFI, Raven's Advanced Progressive Matrices. Family psychiatric history was assessed by participants checking presence or absence of 25 possible DSMIV-TR mental illnesses 'that you know have affected any members of your family'. | 6 verbal creativity tasks and 8 drawing creativity tasks. | • Two factors were obtained: a 'positive schizotypy'; and a 'negative schizotypy' factor.
• Only intelligence (Raven) and openness (NEO-FFI) predicted verbal creativity in multiple regression.
• Openness predicted drawing creativity even more strongly than it predicts verbal creativity, whereas intelligence predicted drawing creativity significantly, but less strongly than it predicted verbal creativity in multiple regression.
• Self-reported capacities to be creative, inventive, imaginative, interesting, entertaining, funny, and witty were slightly correlated with positive schizotypy.
• Drawing creativity was positively predicted by the family mood/anxiety/personality disorders factor, and negatively predicted by the family impulse control disorders factor. |
| (Preti and Vellante, 2007) | 80 creative artists (CA) and 80 noncreative controls (NC). | Annett Hand Preference Questionnaire, Peters et al. Delusions Inventory, General Health Questionnaire. | 30 musicians, 25 painters, and 25 writers. | • CA were more likely to use the left hand, with more left hand use reported by artists involved in music and painting.
• CA scored higher on the Peters et al. Delusions Inventory.
• CA were more likely to have experienced both licit and illicit psychotropic substances. |

Study	Sample	Design/Measures	Measures	Results
(Forgeard, 2008)	30 authors (10 bipolar disorder, 10 unipolar depression, 10 controls).	Retrospective on biographies.	Linguistic Inquiry and Word Count.	• Bipolar writers referred to death more than did unipolar writers. • Unipolar writers referred to people other than themselves more than did control writers. • Unipolar writers used more words describing cognitive mechanisms (e.g., understand, know) than did both other groups.
(Nelson and Rawlings, 2008)	100 artists (57 females, 43 males).	Big Five Inventory, Unusual Experiences Questionnaire from O-LIFE, Boundary Questionnaire, General Behaviour Inventory.	Experience of Creativity Questionnaire (ECQ).	• Schizotypy (O-LIFE) displayed correlations with all the ECQ scales, apart from Clarity/Preparation.
(Claridge and McDonald, 2009)	77 university students (44 females, 33 males).	O-LIFE, AQ.	Sub-tests from the Wallach–Kogan divergent thinking test, two convergent thinking tasks: Missionaries and Cannibals, and Tower of Hanoi.	• Suggested relationships between negative schizotypy, autistic traits, and convergent thinking. • Expected association between positive schizotypy and divergent thinking was not replicated.
(C. Murphy, 2009)	Salvador Dalí.	Presence of psychotic disorder (OPCRIT) and personality disorder questionnaire (PDQ-R), retrospectively.	–	• Dalí was found to meet the diagnostic criteria for several DSM Cluster A and Cluster B personality disorders, as well as for psychotic illnesses.

(continued)

Table 6.1 Continued

(Keri, 2009)	200 healthy participants with high intellectual and academic performance. Another 128 participants provided population means for creative tests.	Structured Clinical Interview for DSM-IV, IQ (Wechsler, 1981), and schizotypal traits (SPQ). Genotyping was performed for single-nucleotide polymorphisms of the Neuregulin 1 gene.	CAQ and the 'Just Suppose' subtest of TTCT.	• Neuregulin 1 gene (SNP8NRG243177/rs6994992) is associated with CAQ and TTCT. • Highest creative achievements and creative thinking scores were found in people who carried the T/T genotype, previously shown related to psychosis risk.
(Tremblay et al., 2010)	84 individuals in the sample with information on occupation who have a DSM-III manic episode diagnosis (46 with inpatient treatment).	NIMH Diagnostic Interview Schedule (DIS) for DSM-III. DIS responses were entered into a computer.	Creative occupation.	• Those with bipolar illness appear to be disproportionately concentrated in the most creative occupational category.
(Srivastava et al., 2010)	32 bipolar disorder patients (BP), 21 unipolar major depressive disorder patients (MDD), 22 creative controls (CC), and 42 healthy controls (HC) (all euthymic).	NEO PI-R, TEMPS-A, the Myers-Briggs Type Inventory (MBTI).	BWAS, the Adjective Check List Creative Personality Scale (ACL), and the Figural and Verbal TTCT.	• BP and CC (but not MDD) compared to HC had higher BWAS-Total and BWAS-Dislike scores, and higher MBTI-Intuition preference type rates. • BP, MDD, and CC, compared to HC, had increased TEMPS-A-Cyclothymia scores, and NEO-Neuroticism scores. • NEO-Neuroticism and TEMPS-A Cyclothymia correlated with BWAS-Dislike (and BWAS-Total). • MBTI-Intuition continuous scores and NEO-Openness correlated with BWAS-Like (and BWAS-Total).

(Rybakowski and Klonowska, 2011)	40 patients with bipolar disorder (BP), and 48 controls.	ICD-10 and DSM-IV criteria. Hamilton Depression Rating Scale (HDRS), Young Mania Rating Scale (YMRS), Schizotypy (O-LIFE).	Revised Art Scale (RAS) based on BWAS, test battery 'inventiveness' of the Berlin Intelligence Structure Test (BIS).	• BP better results on the total creativity BIS scale and also on a BIS subscale of verbal creativity. • Detrimental effect of depression on creativity measured by the BIS scale. • In BP, the total O-LIFE correlated with RAS-like, RAS-dislike and RAS total. • Impulsive Nonconformity in O-LIFE correlated with BIS.
(Kyaga et al., 2011)	54042 people with schizophrenia (SZ), 29 644 people with bipolar disorder (BP) and 217 771 people with unipolar depression (UD). First-, second-, and third-degree relatives of these individuals were also included. Ten matched controls for each person in the case group and each of their relatives.	ICD8-10.	Creative professions (artistic and scientific).	• Individuals with BP and healthy siblings of people with SZ or BP were overrepresented in creative professions. • People with schizophrenia had no increased rate of overall creative professions compared with controls, but an increased rate in the subgroup of artistic occupations.
(Soeiro-de-Souza et al., 2011)	67 bipolar type I patients. 20 patients were experiencing manic episodes; 21 mixed states and 26 depressive episodes.	Structured Clinical Interview (SCID-I/P) for DSM-IV TR. The Young Mania Rating Scale (YMRS), and the Montgomery–Asberg Depression Rating Scale (MADRS), Clinical Global Impression scale, Wisconsin Card Sorting Test (WCST), Wechsler Abbreviated Scale of Intelligence (WASI).	BWAS.	• Manic and mixed state patients had higher creativity scores than depressive individuals. • Creativity was influenced by executive function measures only in manic patients. • Intelligence did not influence creativity for any of the mood episode types.

(continued)

Table 6.1 Continued

(Vellante et al., 2011)	152 undergraduate creative students and 152 students in areas mainly requiring application of learned rules.	TEMPS-A, the General Health Questionnaire (GHQ).	CAQ.	• Creative people scored higher than controls on the CAQ and on the cyclothymic, hyperthymic and irritable subscales of the TEMPS-A. • CAQ was positively associated with cyclothymic and hyperthymic, and partly with irritable subscales of the TEMPS-A.
(Fink et al., 2012)	69 participants (18 Alcohol dependents, 18 polysubstance dependents, 21 university students, 17 actors).	EPQ, Brief Symptom Inventory, Wonderlic Personnel Test, Latent inhibition (LI).	Berliner Intelligenz Struktur Test, Picture Completion subtest of the TTCT.	• Actors and polydrug dependents had high scores on psychoticism, high originality during creative idea generation, and decreased LI as compared with the other groups. • Associations between LI, originality, and psychoticism were found.
(Soeiro-de-Souza et al., 2012)	66 medication-free subjects with bipolar disorder (BD) (41 in manic and 25 in depressive episodes) and 78 healthy controls.	Diagnosis was determined by psychiatrists using the Structured Clinical Interview (SCID-I) for DSM-IV TR. Mini International Neuropsychiatric Interview, Young Mania Rating Scale, Montgomery–Asberg Depression Rating Scale, neurocognitive tests for attention, verbal memory, visuospatial function, language, psychomotor speed, executive function, and intelligence. Genotyped for BDNF Val66Met.	BWAS.	• Manic patients with the Val allele (Met−) had higher BWAS scores than Met+ carriers. • This relationship was not observed among patients in depressive episodes or among control subjects.

Study	Sample	Diagnostic criteria	Measures	Findings
(Kyaga et al., 2012)	1173763 patients with schizophrenia, schizoaffective disorder, bipolar disorder, unipolar depression, anxiety disorders, alcohol abuse, drug abuse, autism, ADHD, anorexia nervosa, and completed suicide. First-, second-, and third-degree relatives of these individuals were also included. Ten matched controls for each person in the case group and each of their relatives.	ICD8-10.	Creative professions (artistic and scientific).	• Except for bipolar disorder, individuals with overall creative professions were not more likely to suffer from investigated psychiatric disorders than controls. • Authors were specifically associated with increased likelihood of schizophrenia, bipolar disorder, unipolar depression, anxiety disorders, substance abuse, and suicide. • There was an association between overall creative professions and first-degree relatives of patients with schizophrenia, bipolar disorder, anorexia nervosa, and for siblings of patients with autism.
(Jaracz et al., 2012)	43 patients with paranoid schizophrenia in symptomatic remission and 45 healthy controls.	A consensus diagnosis of paranoid schizophrenia was made for each patient, by at least two psychiatrists, according to DSM-IV criteria. Patients with a total positive and negative symptoms scale (PANSS) score of less than 60 were included.	BWAS and the inventiveness part of the Berlin Intelligence Structure Test (BIS). Executive functions were measured by means of the Wisconsin Card Sorting Test (WCST).	• Patients gave responses on the BWAS, had lower total score on the BIS and in the figural test, and performed worse on all domains of the WCST compared with controls. • Their lower scores on the BIS correlated with lower scores on the WCST.
(Young et al., 2013)	2482 15- to 16-year-old adolescents.	Center for Epidemiological Studies Depression Scale (CES-D).	Amount of involvement in arts and sports in the time period after school, verbal IQ (Peabody Picture Vocabulary Test–Revised), working memory (Wechsler Intelligence Scales for Children–Revised).	• Teens involved in afterschool arts had higher depressive symptom scores than those not involved. • The association between arts involvement and depressive symptoms held only for those scoring above the median in working memory.

Table 6.2 Summary of studies primarily investigating neurodevelopmental disorders

Reference	Study sample	Assessment of mental disorder	Definition of creativity	Findings
(Argulewicz et al., 1979)	39 elementary grade children.	Diagnosed as learning disabled.	TTCT, Figural form A.	• Scored in the same range as average children on all constructs of creativity except elaboration. On this component they scored below average.
(Sigg and Gargiulo, 1980)	42 learning disabled and 44 nondisabled students. Mean chronological age for the learning disabled students was 9.4 and 8.8 for nondisabled learners.	Handicapped learners were chosen from self-contained special education classrooms.	Matching Familiar Figures Test and the TTCT.	• Learning disabled and nondisabled students did not significantly differ in their performance on the TTCT.
(Graham and Sheinker, 1980)	26 learning-disabled and 30 average students in grades 3, 4, and 5.	Learning-disabled students were receiving services in a program for perceptual communication.	Figural Form A of the TTCT and Sounds and Images, containing a series of free-association tasks designed to measure originality.	• Learning-disabled and average students produced equivalent numbers of relevant responses on nonverbal measures of creativity. • Learning-disabled students were less able to generate new ideas and change an initial approach.
(Eisen, 1989)	Sixteen normally performing and 16 children with learning disabilities (LD) were administered a non-verbal creativity task and a control task of verbal fluency. The age of the subjects ranged from 8 years, 5 months to 11 years, 11 months.	All the LD students had been diagnosed by the Chicago public school system.	Assorted geometric shapes were used as test items. The subjects were asked to create pictures from these shapes. These pictures were in turn scored on their originality, remoteness, and fluency.	• Children with LD scored higher on the nonverbal but not the verbal control task. • Increased performances of children with learning disabilities were found in remoteness, originality, and number of pieces per picture.

Study	Subjects	Diagnosis	Measures	Results
(Funk et al., 1993)	19 boys with ADHD and 21 comparison boys aged 8 through 11. Boys with ADHD received prescribed methylphenidate only for the first session.	ADHD must have been previously determined by physician or multidisciplinary team diagnosis, the child must have been currently receiving methylphenidate therapy, and there must have been elevations in Conners' Hyperactivity Index score by parent report.	Alternate forms of the TTCT- Figural (nonverbal). Two administrations of tests of creativity.	• Mean Torrance summary scores for comparison boys were higher than for boys with ADHD. • No changes in performance over medication state (ADHD group) were observed.
(Turner, 1999)	Four groups of subjects: high-functioning (IQ>75) with autism (HFA; n = 22), high-functioning controls (HFC; n = 22), autism (LDA; n = 22), learning disabled controls (LDC; n = 22). Subjects were aged 6-32 years.	Diagnoses were verified at the time of the study through two interviews administrated incorporating diagnostic criteria for autism outlined in the DSM-III-R.	Letter fluency task, Category fluency task, Uses of objects task, Pattern meaning task, Design fluency task	• Subjects with autism showed reduced fluency for both word and ideational fluency tasks. • The design fluency paradigm revealed no significant difference in the quantity of designs generated, but a clear qualitative difference. The autistic group produced higher rates of disallowed and perseverative responses.
(Healey and Rucklidge, 2005)	67 children, ages 10 to 12 (33 ADHD and 34 controls). 30 of ADHD children were taking medication (methylphenidate). They were asked not to take it 24 hrs prior to the day of testing.	ADHD was diagnosed by a psychiatrist or registered psychologist. Parent and teacher forms of the Conners' Rating Scales-Revised.	TTCT Figural form A, Maier's Two-String Problem, and the Block Design and Vocabulary subsets of the Wechsler Intelligence Scale for Children (WISC-III).	• No significant difference between the ADHD group's and control group's performance on either the TTCT, Maier's Two-String Problem, or WISC-III.

(continued)

Table 6.2 Continued

(Abraham et al., 2006)	11 ADHD (3 girls, 8 boys) patients, 12 patients with conduct disorder (CD) (4 girls, 8 boys), and a control group of 21 children (9 girls, 12 boys) who had no history of mental illness.	3 IQ subscales (Verbal Factor, Reasoning, and Closure) from the Leistungsprüfsystem. Patients were diagnosed using DSM-IV and recruited with the guidance of the chief consultant psychiatrist from a local Child and Adolescent Psychiatry Unit.	• The ADHD group exhibited an enhanced ability in overcoming the constraining influence of examples, but a reduced capacity to generate a functional invention during the imagery task. • The CD group exhibited poorer performance on the originality component of the creative imagery task in comparison to the control group.
(Healey and Rucklidge, 2006)	29 ADHD children without creativity, 12 creative children (CC) with ADHD symptoms, 18 creative children without ADHD symptoms, and 30 controls.	Parent form of the Conners' Rating Scales-Revised (CPRS-R), K-SADS-PL, Wechsler intelligence scale for children (WISC-III), Rapid Automatized Naming (RAN), Stop task tracking version, Stroop Task, Stroop negative priming task, Tower of London .	• 40% of CC displayed ADHD symptomatology, but none met full criteria for ADHD.
(White and Shah, 2006)	90 university undergraduates (45 ADHD; mean age 19.4 years, 45 controls; mean age 19.5 years).	DSM-IV, Current Symptoms and Childhood Symptoms Scales, Boatwright-Bracken Adult Attention Deficit Disorder Scale. No medication within two weeks prior to participation.	• ADHD individuals outperformed non-ADHD individuals on the Unusual Uses Task. • ADHD individuals performed worse than non-ADHD on the Remote Associates Test and the semantic IOR task.
(Wei, 2011)	127 children with Tourette's Syndrome (TS; 21 females, 106 males; 6 to 12 years) and 138 controls.	DSM-IV criteria, parents' questionnaire of 'School and Family Adjustment'.	• TS had significantly lower scores on Elaboration in the creativity assessment.

(Column 3 task note for White and Shah: RAT, Unusual Uses Task, Semantic Inhibition of Return Task.)

(Column 3 task note for Abraham: Conceptual expansion task, the recently activated knowledge task, the creative imagery task, and the alternate uses task.)

(Column 3 task note for Healey and Rucklidge: TTCT, Maier's two-string problem.)

(Column 3 task note for Wei: Williams's Creativity Assessment Packet of Divergent Thinking Test.)

(White and Shah, 2011)	60 university undergraduates (30 ADHD, 30 controls).	DSM-IV, Current Symptoms and Childhood Symptoms Scales, Conners' adult ADHD rating scale. One half of the ADHD group was taking medication to treat ADHD.	CAQ, FourSight Thinking Profile, Abbreviated Torrance Test for Adults.	• Higher overall creative achievement in the ADHD group. • Adults with ADHD produced more original responses on the verbal component of the Abbreviated Torrance Test for Adults (ATTA).
(Campbell and Wang, 2012)	Online survey of incoming class of 2014 at Princeton University (n = 1077).	Question: 'Do you have a sibling with autism spectrum disorder (ASD)? ASD includes autism, Asperger's, and pervasive developmental disorder not otherwise specified.	527 technical major (natural sciences, engineering, or mathematics), 394 nontechnical majors (245 in social sciences, 149 in humanities), and 156 students were undecided.	• Students aspiring to technical majors were more likely than other students to report a sibling with ASD. • Students interested in the humanities were more likely to report a family member with major depressive, bipolar disorder, or substance abuse problems.
(Pring et al., 2012)	9 savant artists with autism spectrum disorder (SASD), 9 non-talented comparison adults with autism spectrum disorder (ASD), 9 non-talented adults with mild/moderate learning Difficulties (MLD), and 9 artistically talented students.	Peabody Picture Vocabulary Test (PPVT), Raven's Standard Progressive Matrices or Coloured Progressive Matrices.	Incomplete and repeated figures tasks of the TTCT, figural synthesis task (FST).	• On the TTCT, the art students performed significantly better than the other three groups. • SASD produced more elaborate responses than the ASD and MLD groups. • On the non-drawing construction task, SASD produced more original outputs than the ASD, MLD and art student groups.
(Jolley et al., 2013)	60 5-19-year-olds (15 with non-savant autism (AUT) and the others with learning difficulty (MLD), similar mental age (MA) or similar chronological age (CA).	Diagnosed by a fully qualified clinical psychologist according to the DSM criteria.	Happy and sad drawings were requested.	• AUT did not draw fewer people, but more immature forms than mental age controls. • There was tentative evidence that fewer social scenes were produced by AUT.

(continued)

Table 6.2 Continued

(Hobson et al., 2013)	Age- and language-matched children with autism (n = 27), autism spectrum disorder (n = 14), and developmental disorders without autism (n = 16).	Autism Diagnostic Observation Schedule-General and previous clinical diagnoses.	Test of Pretend Play (ToPP), with an additional rating of 'playful pretense'.	• Children with autism showed less playful pretend than participants with developmental disorders who did not have autism. • Limitations in creative, playful pretend among children with autism relate to their restricted interpersonal communication and engagement.

Table 6.3 Summary of studies primarily investigating substance use/abuse disorders

Reference	Study sample	Assessment of mental disorder	Definition of creativity	Findings
(Lang et al., 1984)	40 male undergraduate social drinkers were assigned to one of four treatments in a balanced placebo design. Those actually receiving alcohol consumed a mixture containing .6 g ~ 0.75 ml of ethanol per kg of body weight.	Pretest instrument, including Multiple Affect Adjective Check List, was administered containing questions about demographic characteristics, routine drinking behaviour, and beliefs about own creativity and alcohol's effects on it.	Figural portion and the Unusual Uses subtest of the TTCT. Verbal portion of the TTCT.	• Minimal effects of beverage manipulations on measured. • Individuals who thought they had received alcohol gave significantly more positive evaluations of their creative.
(Ludwig, 1990)	Biographies of 34 well known, heavy drinking, 20th century writers, artists, composers, and performers.	For the entire pool of subjects, the same type of information was systematically gathered from at least one major, published biography and transposed onto elaborate data collection forms.	Their biographies had received a review in the *New York Times* Book Review from 1965 to 1990.	• Alcohol use proved detrimental to productivity in over 75% of the sample, especially in the latter phases of their drinking careers. • It appeared to provide direct benefit for about 9% of the sample, indirect benefit for 50%.
(Brunke and Gilbert, 1992)	11 male social drinkers participated in a creative writing task under two conditions, alcohol and placebo. Alcohol condition was a high dose with 1.1 ml ethanol/kg bodyweight.	Subjects were tested individually and were randomly assigned to one of the two beverage sequences: alcohol on Day 1 and placebo on Day 2, or placebo on Day 1 and alcohol on Day 2.	Figurative language was scored using a procedure adapted from a manual developed by Barlow et al. (1970) for use in researching metaphor usage.	• Subjects wrote more novel tropes while intoxicated than when sober. • Alcohol condition produced a higher proportion of novel tropes to total tropes. • Subjects wrote more words when intoxicated.

(continued)

Table 6.3 Continued

(Noble et al., 1993)	A battery of creativity tests was administered to 56 families (fathers, mothers, and their pubescent sons) representing three groups. Group A + was comprised of recovering alcoholic fathers with a family history of alcoholism (n = 19). Group NA+ consisted of non-alcoholic fathers with a family history of alcoholism (n = 18). Group NA- was composed of non-alcoholic fathers without a family history of alcoholism (n = 19).	Diagnosis of fathers' alcoholism was made according to DSM-III-R criteria. None of the mothers or sons in the three family groups were alcoholic.	Creativity Personality Scale, the four Origence/Intellectence scales from the Adjective Check List, and the How Do You Think Test. Moreover, fathers and sons received two divergent thinking tests, and mothers rated their sons using a special scale from the Adjective Check List. The Wechsler Adult Intelligence Scale was administered to the fathers and the Wechsler Intelligence Scale for Children-Revised was given to the sons.	• Sons of alcoholics scored significantly lower than the other two groups of boys on the Creative Personality Scale. • Alcoholic fathers and their sons scored higher than the other two groups on the High Origence/Low Intellectence scale (AI). • Sons of alcoholic fathers showed significantly lower scores than the other two groups of boys on the How do you think. • On the two divergent thinking tests, alcoholic fathers performed significantly lower than the two groups of non-alcoholic fathers. Sons of alcoholic fathers showed a similar trend, though it was not significant.
(Lapp et al., 1994)	116 men.	0.0, 1.1, or 2.2 ml 80% vodka -> 0.0, 0.02, or 0.04 ml alcohol/dl blood.	A card-sorting task assessing creative synthesis of emergent relations.	• No pharmacological effect of alcohol on the creative combinations that subjects produced. • Novelty and structural recombination were enhanced when subjects thought they had consumed alcohol.

(Lowe, 1994)	16 social drinkers (8 females, 8 males) performed under 2 conditions, alcohol and a placebo.	Alcohol dose = 0.83 ml ethanol/kg body weight.	Verbal forms of the TTCT.	• Significant group differences in the alcohol-creativity interaction were noted; performance of higher-scoring in the placebo condition; subjects was impaired (mean: 241.9 ->202.7) by alcohol whereas that of lower-scoring subjects was enhanced (mean: 147.1->179.2).
(Plucker and Dana, 1998)	The impact of parental substance abuse problems on 163 undergraduates' creative achievement.	Core Alcohol and Drug Survey. Students also reported whether their parents had substance abuse problems.	Creative Behaviour Inventory.	• Parental alcohol and drug problems did not have an effect on students' creative achievement.
(Schafer et al., 2012)	160 cannabis users were tested on a day when sober and another day when intoxicated with cannabis. Quartile splits compared those lowest (n = 47) and highest (n = 43) in CAQ.	A sample of cannabis was taken to be analysed for levels of THC. Psychotomimetic States Inventory (PSI), Schizotypal Personality Questionnaire (SPQ), Weschler Test of Adult Reading (WTAR), Spielberger Trait Anxiety Inventory (STAI), Severity of Dependence Scale (SDS), Beck Depression Inventory (BDI).	Verbal fluency task, category fluency task, RAT, CAQ.	• Cannabis increased verbal fluency in low creative to the same level as that of high creative. • The high creativity group was significantly higher in trait schizotypy, but this was not linked to the verbal fluency change.
(Jarosz et al., 2012)	40 male social drinkers (20 in the alcohol (A) intoxication condition and 20 in the sober comparison (C) condition).	Operation Span Task (OSpan), alcohol condition (.88 g ~ 1.10 ml /kg body weight).	RAT.	• A solved more RAT problems than their sober counterparts. • This increase in solution success was accompanied by a decrease in time to correct solution for A. • A rated their experience of problem solving as being more insightful.

Table 6.4 Summary of studies primarily investigating neurological disorders

Reference	Study sample	Assessment of mental disorder	Definition of creativity	Findings
(Miller et al., 1998)	69 patients with frontotemporal dementia (FTD. 5 became artists in the early stages of FTD.	Mini-Mental State Examination, Wisconsin Card Sorting, Stroop tasks, modified Rey-Osterrieth Complex Figure Copy, MRI, SPECT, autopsy.	Interview.	• 4 of the 5 patients, who became artists, had the temporal variant of FTD.
(Drago et al., 2006)	A visual artist with Lewy body dementia (LBD).	—	*Study 1* evaluated two paintings of the same subject matter, one painted before the illness and the other after the onset. *Study 2* evaluated a collection of his paintings from the time before illness until the time of ceased painting when he was suffering.	• Study 1 found representational ratings for the picture painted with LBD was lower than the picture painted before development of LBD. • Study 2 found that all the artistic qualities measures temporally declined except novelty.
(De Souza et al., 2010)	17 patients with frontotemporal lobar degeneration (fvFTLD), 12 nondemented Parkinson's disease (PD) patients, and 17 healthy controls.	Revised Lund-Manchester consensus criteria, MRI in all patients, and 13 out 17 patients had a SPECT, MMSE, Frontal Assessment Battery (FAB), Clinical Dementia Rating (CDR), MADRS, Trail Making Test (TMT), Stroop test, modified Wisconsin Card Sorting Test, verbal fluency, Working memory was evaluated with direct and indirect visual and verbal spans, Social and Emotional Assessment (SEA).	TTCT.	• FvFTLD were strongly impaired in all dimensions of the TTCT, compared to PD and controls. • Disinhibited and perseverative responses were observed only in fvFTLD patients. • Poor creativity was positively correlated with several frontal tests. • Poor creativity was also correlated with prefrontal hypoperfusion.

Study	Sample	Methods / Tasks	Results
(Canesi et al., 2012)	36 Parkinson's disease patients with (PD-c) or without (PD-nc) increased artistic-like production and 36 healthy controls (HC).	Diagnosis of PD according to UK Brain Bank criteria. Mini-mental state examination, frontal lobe assessment battery, clock drawing test, Rey figure copy and recall, verbal and phonemic fluency, and Raven matrices. Unified Parkinsons Disease Rating Scale motor score (UPDRS-III) and Hoehn-Yahr staging. Artistic-like productivity was defined to be enhanced if patients reported working on any form of art more than 2 h per day after the introduction of dopaminergic treatment. TTCT, Barratt Impulsiveness Scale (BIS-11A), the Minnesota Impulsive Disorders Interview (MIDI), and the Punding Rating Scale.	• Mean TTCT score of PD-c was found to be similar to HC, and both PD-c and HC had significantly higher TTCT scores than patients with PD-nc. • No correlation was found between TTCT, BIS-11A, and MIDI.
(Abraham et al., 2012)	74 patients recruited from the Neurological Day Clinic database. Healthy control participants (CT) were selected to match each patient.	Patients were examined by the clinic's chief neurologist prior to the study. Lesion sites were determined by MRI and evaluated by an experienced neuroanatomist. Patients had lesions mainly in the frontal lobe (FL; 9 females, 20 males), parietal–temporal lobe (PTL; 1 females, 10 males), or basal ganglia (BG; 4 females, 12 males). Conceptual expansion task, the creative imagery task, the constraints of examples task, the alternate uses task, RAT, and analytical problem solving tasks (insight and incremental).	• PTL and frontolateral groups revealed poorer overall performance with PTL demonstrating problems with fluency measures, whereas the frontolateral were also less proficient at originality. • BG and frontopolar groups demonstrated superior performance in the ability to overcome constraints imposed by salient semantic distractors when generating creative responses.

Table 6.5 Summary of studies investigating other mental disorders

Reference	Study sample	Assessment of mental disorder	Definition of creativity	Findings
(McNeil, 1971)	43 adults adopted by non-biologically related families were compared to 23 non-creative adoptees. The final population consisted of 50 adoptees.	Rates of mental illness were determined among all included subjects and their parents and siblings.	Creative ability was operationally defined by a committee evaluation. The subjects were divided into three groups; high-, above-average-, and low-creative ability.	• Mental illness rates in the adoptees were positively related to their creative abilities. • Mental illness rates of the biological parents were positively related to the creative abilities of the adoptees. • Mental illness rates among adoptive parents were independent of the adoptees' creative abilities.
(Glover and Tramel, 1976)	Students 14-19 yrs. without (n = 200) and with (n = 194) behavioural problems.	Students with behavioural problems had been suspended from school on at least one occasion during the current school year.	Unusual Uses subtest of the TTCT, Verbal Form b.	• Students identified as having behavioural problems scored significantly higher on two components of creative ability, flexibility and originality.
(Paget, 1979)	16 emotionally disturbed pre-schoolers ranging in age from 3 to 6 years.	Data on file for the children were gathered concerning their intelligence, socio-emotional development, and length of time in treatment.	Torrance preschool measure.	• Results suggest that the emotionally disturbed pre-schoolers were as creative as normal pre-schoolers.
(Smith and Carlsson, 1983)	31 psychiatric patients with anxiety and 43 controls.	Interview.	Interview.	• Anxiety did not facilitate creativity in patients as was the case with controls.
(Mraz and Runco, 1994)	81 college students.	Scale for Suicide Ideation (BSSI), Suicide Ideation Scale (SSI), Hopelessness Scale (HS), Suicide Opinion Questionnaire (SOQ), Perceived Stress Scale (PSS), Student Stress Inventory.	Divergent thinking tasks.	• Problem generation scores were significantly correlated (fluency positively, flexibility negatively) with suicide ideation.

(Stack, 1996)	Artists aged 21–64 years (n = ?).	Official suicide statistics.	Artists were defined as authors, musicians, actors, painters, and dancers.	• After controlling for gender and sociodemographic variables, artists had a 125% higher risk of suicide than among non-artists
(Preti and Miotto, 1999)	Artists found in Garzanci's Encyclopaedia (n = 3093).	Suicide, based on all the biographies cited in the two repertoires for eminent people eligible for the study.	1300 writers, 692 poets, 267 dramaturgians and comedians, 210 architects, 531 painters, 93 sculptors.	• Comparison by profession indicates that poets and writers exceed the mean suicide ratio of the sample. • Painters and architects, conversely, have a clearly lower risk than the mean.
(Preti et al., 2001)	The percentage of deaths by suicide in a sample of 4564 eminent artists who died in the 19th and 20th centuries. Of the sample, 2259 were writers, 834 visual artists, and 1471 musicians.	Suicide.	Eminence was defined as a record in Garzanti's Art, Literature, and Music Encyclopaedia.	• 63 suicides in the sample (1.3% of total deaths). • Musicians (0.2%) as a group had lower suicide rates than literary (2.3%) and visual artists (0.7%).
(Chavez-Eakle et al., 2006)	30 with high creative achievement (HC) dedicated to full-time scientific or artistic creation, 30 controls administrative staff and graduate students, 30 psychiatric outpatients.	Temperament and Character Inventory (TCI), Symptom Check List (SCL)–90. Three different psychiatrists confirmed psychiatric diagnosis. Included diagnoses were mainly major depressive disorder and anxiety disorders.	TTCT.	• HC scored low on psychopathology. • There were strong negative correlations between creativity and psychopathology on all subscales.

(continued)

Table 6.5 Continued

(Akinola and Mendes, 2008)	96 young adults (65 females, 31 males).	Saliva sample that assayed for dehydroepiandrosterone (DHEAS), experiment of social approval or social rejection, Positive and Negative Affect Schedule.	Abbreviated Torrance Test for Adults, an artistic creativity Task (CAT).	• Social rejection was associated with greater artistic creativity; however, the interaction between affective vulnerability (lower baseline DHEAS) and condition was significant, suggesting that situational triggers of negative affect were especially influential among those lower in DHEAS, which resulted in the most creative products.
(Silvia and Kimbrel, 2010)	189 university students (150 females, 39 males).	Depression and Anxiety subscales of the Depression Anxiety Stress Scales, Social Interaction Anxiety Scale.	3 divergent thinking tasks, 9-item Creativity Scale for Different Domains, Creative Behaviour Inventory, Creative Achievement Questionnaire.	• Overall, measures of anxiety, depression, and social anxiety predicted little variance in creativity. Few models explained more than 3% of the variance.

and paranoid thoughts), negative schizotypy (e.g., social isolation and reduced emotional expression), and cognitive disorganization (e.g., poor attention and concentration as well as poor decision-making) (Claridge et al., 1996; Mason and Claridge, 2006). To the extent that studies report an association for schizotypy with creativity, these are consistent with *positive* schizotypy. Related to investigations of subsyndromal symptoms being related to creativity, a few studies have also investigated non-diagnosed relatives of patients with either schizophrenia or bipolar disorder, often demonstrating increased creative abilities in these individuals. The underlying assumption is that relatives of patients share traits but display lower symptom severity, which might be more advantageous for creativity than the fulminant disorder (Richards et al., 1988).

Schizophrenia

Patients with schizophrenia Many of the early studies reviewed are aimed at schizophrenia. In general, studies have failed to establish increased creative abilities in patients with schizophrenia. For example, in 1959 Herbert had already described a group of 60 patients, including those with schizophrenia, admitted from 1928 to 1955 (1959). He could find no increased rate of artistic occupations in the group. Andreasen and Powers observed both patients with schizophrenia and bipolar disorder (1974), showing that patients with schizophrenia tended to be over-inclusive and demonstrating less richness and bizarreness in writing, compared to the writers and those with a history of mania in the same study. Comparable results were received by Dykes and Mcghie who concluded that schizophrenic patients' widening of attention was without intention and resulted in creative performance being hindered (1976). Patients with schizophrenia have also been demonstrated to perform worse on the RAT, and other creative tests compared to healthy controls (Abraham et al., 2007; Folley and Park, 2005). Thus, Abraham et al. concluded that there was no apparent negative correlation between cognitive control and creative abilities. Jaracz et al. confirmed the latter by demonstrating that lower scores on the inventiveness part of the Berlin Intelligence Structure Test positively correlated with lower scores on the Wisconsin Card Sorting Test (2012). We found no support for a higher incidence of creative professions among patients with schizophrenia in two nation-wide studies of schizophrenic patients compared to healthy controls; however, there was a significant increase in people with artistic occupations (Kyaga et al., 2012; Kyaga et al., 2011). Studies exploring prominent personalities have rarely found a greater proportion of schizophrenia among them.

Andreasen, for example, examined 30 creative writers and found many of them suffering from affective disorders, but none afflicted with schizophrenia (1987).

Psychoticism and schizotypy   Although few studies have linked schizophrenia *disorder* and creative abilities, several studies have found an association between subsyndromal psychotic symptoms (psychoticism or schizotypy), with creativity. Kidner was able to show such a relationship between EPQ and the originality and fluency scores from a creative index (1976). Kline and Cooper found a similar relationship between EPQ and verbal fluency, but in males only (1986). Schuldberg et al. demonstrated a correlation between positive schizotypy and creativity as measured by the BWAS and How do you think (1988). Similar findings were made by Kinney et al. using the Lifetime Creativity Scales (2000), and Weinstein and Graves using the Remote Associate Test and a written fluency test (2002). Folley et al. found heightened divergent thinking capacity in schizotypal subjects compared to both healthy controls and patients with schizophrenia (Folley and Park, 2005). By using near-infrared optical spectroscopy, these authors proposed that the increased ability in divergent thinking was concurrent with activation of the right prefrontal cortex. Similar suggestions had been done in the study by Weinstein and Graves referenced above (2002). In a more comprehensive study of 425 British adults (269 females, 156 males), positive schizotypy, evaluated by *unusual experiences* in the O-LIFE inventory, was positively correlated with mating success mediated through accomplishment in creative activities (Nettle and Clegg, 2006). Nettle also showed that while poets and artists were similar to schizophrenic patients with regards to unusual experiences, they exhibited less *introvertive anhedonia*, i.e., negative schizotypy, compared to patients with schizophrenia (Nettle, 2006). Similar findings of O-LIFE and creativity were made by Burch et al. (2006), although Claridge et al. were unable to replicate the correlation between positive schizotypy and divergent thinking (2009). Nelson and Rawlings were able to demonstrate an association between a phenomenological approach to creativity and O-LIFE (2008). Finally, Miller and Tal using another inventory for schizotypy (Schizotypal Personality Questionnaire) in 225 university students again concluded that there were significant associations between positive schizotypy, and verbal and drawing creativity (2007). However, the increase in creative abilities was suggested to be mediated by the Big five personality trait of *openness to experience*.

Relatives to patients with schizophrenia   Concurrent with studies of subsyndromal psychotic symptoms rather than fulminant schizophrenia, some authors have explored non-diagnosed relatives of patients with schizophrenia. Among the first was Karlsson, who through investigating books on genealogy published by different authors and covering all regions of Iceland, demonstrated that relatives (n = 486) of patients with schizophrenia were more often found in *Who's Who* compared to the general population (1970). Given that certain branches were high in both psychosis and listings in *Who's Who*, the author concluded that findings were probably due to shared genetics. Similar ideas were also advanced in the study by Keri, who in 200 healthy individuals demonstrated that a variant of the Neuregulin 1 gene (see Chapter 5), related to increased psychosis risk, was correlated with the CAQ and the Just suppose subtest of the TTCT (2009). Karlsson followed up his own results in a study of 8007 relatives to persons with psychosis, and found that these were more often authors of published books than the general population (1984). A considerable smaller study by Kauffmann et al. on the six most socially and intellectually competent children of mothers with schizophrenia and other psychiatric disorders, concluded that these children were more creative compared to controls (1979). Finally, our two nation-wide studies results affirmed an increase in, not only artistic occupations, but also overall creative professions (artistic and scientific occupations), in healthy first-degree relatives of patients with schizophrenia (Kyaga et al., 2013; Kyaga et al., 2011).

Bipolar disorder

Patients with bipolar disorder   Whereas few studies have provided results supporting an association between schizophrenia disorder and creativity, the reverse can be said about mood disorders and especially bipolar disorder. One of the most well-known studies was completed by Andreasen investigating 30 creative writers active at the Iowa writers' workshop, as well as the writers' first-degree relatives (1987). The Iowa workshop is one of the most widely recognized creative-writing programmes in the United States. Eighty per cent of the writers, compared to 30 per cent of controls, were found to have been suffering an affective disorder sometime in their lives. A high proportion of the writers suffered from bipolar disorder (writers: 43 per cent vs. controls: 10 per cent). Jamison correspondingly investigated 47 British writers and artists, reporting that 38 per cent had been treated for an affective illness (1989). The playwrights had the highest overall rate (63 per cent) of an affective illness, but only poets had been treated with more serious interventions, such as hospitalization, lithium, ECT, etc. for bipolar illness. Ludwig likewise established an increased rate of manic episodes in a group of just over 1000 individuals based on their biographies having been published in the *New York Times* book review from 1960 to 1990 (1992, 1995). This increase was even further pronounced when only those active within classical creative professions were included (~3 per cent vs. ~10 per cent). Post investigated 291 world-famous men in science, thought, politics, and art, establishing an increase in depressive conditions, with psychoses entirely restricted to affective varieties (1994). Again, writers were especially struck by psychopathology with a total of 72 per cent having experienced a mood episode. Post then followed up his study with another study of about 100 well-known diseased British and American prose and play writers (1996), reporting psychopathology within the affective spectrum in 80.0 per cent of poets, 80.5 per cent of novelists/poets, and in 87.5 per cent of playwrights. Richards et al. investigated patients with bipolar disorder, cyclothymes, and relatives of patients using the Lifetime Creativity Scales (1988). Results failed to show an increase of creativity in only patients vs. controls, but there was an increase in the combined group of patients and relatives vs. controls. Simeonova et al. studied 40 adults with bipolar disorder, 20 bipolar offspring with bipolar disorder, 20 bipolar offspring with ADHD, and 18 healthy control parents and their 18 healthy control children using the BWAS (2005). Patients were diagnosed by using the Structured Clinical Interview for DSM-IV Axis I Disorders. Results revealed that adults with bipolar disorder compared to controls scored (120 per cent) higher on the BWAS Dislike subscale. Mean BWAS Dislike subscale scores were also higher in offspring with bipolar disorder (107 per cent higher) and offspring with ADHD (91 per cent higher) than in healthy control children. These results were joined by a study performed by Santosa et al., in which patients with bipolar disorder and creative controls, but not patients with major depressive disorder, scored significantly higher on total BWAS compared to normal controls (2007). We investigated patients receiving psychiatric inpatient treatment, and demonstrated a significant increased occurrence of overall creative professions in bipolar disorder, but not in major depressive disorder (Kyaga et al., 2011). These results were later confirmed in the follow-up study, where outpatient-treated patients were also included (Kyaga et al., 2013).

A particular inquiry related to creativity and bipolar disorder has been the impact of lithium treatment. Lithium has been the gold standard for treating bipolar disorder since the 1970s and remains the gold standard today (Hirschowitz et al., 2010; Schou et al., 1971).

However, it is suggested that heightened creativity during hypomanic episodes may contribute to ambivalence about seeking treatment or undermine adherence to treatment (American Psychiatric Association and American Psychiatric Association. DSM-5 Task Force, 2013). Three studies investigate lithium in relation to creativity specifically, although only two provide clear results. Shaw et al. examined the effect of lithium on the productivity and idiosyncrasy of written associations in 22 euthymic outpatients with affective disorder (1986). Lithium discontinuation produced a significant increase in associational productivity and idiosyncrasy, while restoration of lithium dosage reversed both these effects. On the other hand, Schou interviewed 24 'manic depressive' artists with lithium treatment about their creative abilities during treatment, and most (n = 12) reported favourable effects on artistic productivity in the long run (1979).

The affective temperament A few studies have addressed the affective temperament in relation to creative behaviour. For example, Strong et al. demonstrated that *cyclothymia* and *dysthymia* assessed by the Temperament evaluation of the Memphis, Pisa, Paris and San Diego autoquestionnaire (TEMPS-A) was correlated to BWAS Total scores and BWAS Dislike subscale scores (2007). Srivastava et al. have shown that bipolar disorder, major depressive disorder, and creative controls, compared to normal controls, display increased TEMPS-A cyclothymia scores (2010). Likewise, Vellante et al. demonstrated that undergraduate students attending preparatory courses for creative artistic professions scored higher on the cyclothymic, hyperthymic and irritable subscales of the TEMPS-A, while scores on the CAQ was positively correlated with cyclothymic and hyperthymic, and partly with irritable subscales of the TEMPS-A (2011).

Relatives to patients with bipolar disorder Studies of relatives to patients with bipolar disorder have also revealed interesting results. About a quarter (n = 124) of the index patients in Karlsson's study on 487 relatives of patients with psychosis were 'manic depressives' (1970). In Richards and co-workers' study exploring patients with bipolar disorder, cyclothymia, and relatives to patients using the Lifetime Creativity Scales, results indicated higher creativity among healthy relatives of patients than among 'manic depressives' (p<.10) (1988). As stated previously, in the study by Simeonova et al. mean BWAS Dislike subscale scores were higher in bipolar disorder offspring with bipolar disorder (107 per cent higher) and bipolar disorder offspring with ADHD (91 per cent higher) than in healthy control children (2005). Finally, in our studies; non-diagnosed first-degree relatives of patients with bipolar disorder generally demonstrated similar increases, as the patients in the occurrence of creative professions compared to controls (Kyaga et al., 2012; Kyaga et al., 2011).

Neurodevelopmental disorders

Although far fewer studies have examined neurodevelopmental disorders than psychotic and mood disorders concerning creativity, there has been a considerable interest in whether young patients with these disorders have creative abilities exceeding those of their peers. Most studies have included learning disabled children and students. Lately, focus has shifted to ADHD and possible effects of medication in these disorders.

Autism spectrum disorders

Turner examined individuals aged 6–32 years who were high-functioning (IQ>75) with autism (n = 22), high-functioning controls (n = 22), autistic (n = 22), and learning disabled controls (n = 22) (1999). Subjects with autism generally showed reduced fluency for both words and ideation. Another study by Pring et al. included 9 savant artists with autism spectrum disorder (SASD), 9 non-talented comparison adults with autism spectrum disorder (ASD), 9 non-talented adults with mild/moderate learning difficulties (MLD), and 9 artistically talented students (2012). Results demonstrated that the art students performed superior to the other three groups on the TTCT, while SASD made more elaborate responses than the ASD and MLD groups on a drawing task. On a non-drawing construction task, SASD made more original creations than the ASD, MLD and art student groups. We found that while patients with autism were not overrepresented in creative professions, the opposite was true for non-diagnosed siblings of patients (Kyaga et al., 2012). This increase was especially pronounced in the subgroup of scientific occupations. However, both parents and offspring to patients in this study demonstrated no comparable increase in creative professions. Campbell and Wang made an online survey of an incoming class to Princeton University and reported that students aspiring for *technical majors* were more likely than other students to have a sibling with ASD (2012).

ADHD

In line with the rising awareness on ADHD (ADHD-Awareness-Month, 2014), some authors have explored whether there is any connection between ADHD and creative capabilities. Funk et al. investigated 19 boys with previously diagnosed ADHD and 21 comparison boys aged 8 to 11 on two administrations of TTCT-Figural (nonverbal) (Funk et al., 1993). Boys with ADHD were given methylphenidate (standard pharmacological treatment for ADHD) only for the first session. Creativity scores for comparison boys were somewhat higher than for boys with ADHD. No changes in performance across medication state were observed. Healey and Rucklidge investigated 67 children, ages 10 to 12 (33 patients with ADHD unmedicated for 24hr, and 34 controls), finding no significant difference between the ADHD group's and control group's performances on creativity scores (2005). In a second study, Healey et al. demonstrated that 40 per cent of a sample of creative children displayed ADHD symptomatology, but none met full criteria for ADHD (2006). Abraham et al. found that ADHD patients displayed a reduced capacity to create an invention during an imagery task (2006). Likewise, we could not find any evidence of increased occurrence of creative occupations in patients with ADHD or their relatives (Kyaga et al., 2012). White and Shah on the other hand, reported in two studies that university undergraduates with ADHD scored higher on both divergent thinking measures and creative achievements (2006, 2011). Also, in the previously cited study by Simeonova et al., mean creativity scores assessed by the BWAS Dislike subscale were also higher in a subgroup of offspring to patients with bipolar disorder diagnosed with ADHD compared to healthy control children (2005).

Learning disability disorders

Studies of creativity in individuals with learning disability disorders have a longer history than for ADHD. Argulewicz et al. studied 39 elementary grade children with learning disability in 1979. These children scored as average children on all constructs of creativity except *elaboration*, where they scored significantly below average. Comparable results were found by Sigg et al. and Graham et al., who reported that children with learning disability disorders scored similar or below average on different aspects of creativity (Graham and Sheinker, 1980; Sigg and Gargiulo, 1980). Eisen conversely reported increased performance of 16 children with learning disabilities administered a nonverbal creativity task compared to controls (1989). However, the author also reported a negative correlation between the verbal and nonverbal tests, suggesting that there is a link between the verbal deficits and the creative style of children with learning disabilities.

Substance use/abuse

Beveridge and Yorston contended that while the medical establishment largely takes a negative view on alcohol use and especially abuse, the opposite is true for the lay public and many writers and artists (1999). They value alcohol for its ability to make new creative insights, and courageous drinking has long been associated with artistic personality. Rather than being a sign of personal failing, alcoholism is taken as evidence of true artistic integrity. Studies investigating this substance use and abuse in relation to creativity have generally approached the question in two ways. The first is to investigate the direct effect on the creative process of being intoxicated, while the second is to study the effects on creative productivity in the long run under excessive drinking and drug abuse.

Alcohol use/abuse

Brunke and Gilbert told 11 male social drinkers to perform a creative-writing task under alcohol (1.1 ml ethanol/kg body weight) and placebo conditions (1992). All subjects participated in both conditions. Results revealed an absolute increase of novel tropes, as well as the quota of novel tropes compared to total tropes in the alcohol condition. In addition, subjects penned more words when intoxicated. Jarosz et al. similarly found that individuals intoxicated with alcohol (0.88 g ~ 1.10 ml/kg body weight) solved more problems on the RAT than their sober counterparts (Jarosz et al., 2012). Lowe extended these findings in a study of 16 social drinkers performing under alcohol (0.83 ml/kg body weight) and placebo condition (1994). The creative performance of subjects scoring low on creativity in the placebo condition was enhanced by alcohol, whereas those scoring high in creativity during the placebo condition were conversely compromised in creative performance by alcohol. Lang et al. employed a comparable lower dose of alcohol (0.6 g ~ 0.75 ml/kg body weight) with negligible effects on the Figural portion and the Unusual uses subtest of the Verbal portion of the TTCT (1984). Yet, those individuals who thought they had received alcohol gave more positive evaluations of their creative abilities than did subjects who thought they were in the non-alcohol group. Comparable results were reported by Lapp et al. in subjects receiving lower doses of alcohol (max 0.4 ml/kg body weight) (1994).

While studies on alcohol intoxication suggest an advantage for the creative process, studies on excessive alcohol intake in the long run provide more mixed results. Ludwig's study on 1005 exceptional individuals who had their biographies published in the *New York Times* book review from 1960 to 1990 found a general increase in alcohol abuse in artists (1992, 1995). Comparable results were suggested by Post in his study of 291 world-famous men and 100 well-known prose and play writers (Post, 1994, 1996). Again, writers tend to stand out from other artists, further suggested by the results of the study by Andreasen on writers in the Iowa writer's workshop (1987). Thirty per cent of the writers had alcohol abuse compared to 7 per cent of the controls. Then again, when Ludwig investigated the writers in his previous cohort specifically, alcohol use proved detrimental to productivity in more than three-quarters of the sample, especially in the later stages of their drinking careers (1990). Alcoholic fathers compared to non-alcoholic fathers achieved significantly lower scores on divergent thinking tests in a study by Noble et al. (1993). Comparable results were suggested in the sons of these fathers. Plucker and Dana could not validate these findings in a larger group, but did not find any appreciable effect on students' creative achievement related to parental alcohol and drug problems (1998). Finally, our nation-wide study demonstrated a decreased likelihood of holding overall creative professions in patients with alcohol abuse as well as in their relatives (Kyaga et al., 2012). The exception was again found in writers; there was a significant increased occurrence of authors to suffer alcohol abuse compared to controls.

Drug use/abuse

One study tested the impact of cannabis use on creativity (Schafer et al., 2012). Regular cannabis users were submitted to testing on a day when sober and then again another day when under the influence of cannabis. Results demonstrated that cannabis increased verbal fluency in individuals with low creativity in the non-intoxicated phase to the same level as that of individuals with high creativity. No effect on creativity was found in those individuals scoring high on creativity during the non-intoxicated phase. Ludwig's study on 1005 prominent individuals suggested that those active within creative arts more often were drug abusers than the general population (1992, 1995). This could not be validated in our study, which reported that those with drug abuse and their relatives had a decreased occurrence of creative professions (Kyaga et al., 2012). Again, the opposite was true for writers, with authors and their parents having an increased occurrence of drug abuse.

Neurological disorders

Five studies investigated the effects of neurological disease on creativity. These studies have been suggested to especially aid further understanding of the neurophysiology of creativity.

Dementias, Parkinson's disease and other neurological disorders

Miller et al. interviewed 69 patients with frontotemporal dementia (FTD) regarding their visual capabilities (1998). Five of the patients turned to artistic activities in their early disease. These all had the temporal variant of FTD, and the authors therefore suggested that loss of function in the anterior temporal lobes could lead to 'facilitation' of artistic skills. De Souza et al. later demonstrated that individuals with frontotemporal lobar degeneration with severe *frontal* degeneration (fvFTLD) were heavily compromised in all dimensions of the Torrance tests of creative thinking (2010). The authors put forth that any appearance of artistic talent in patients with fvFTLD would be explained by the release of unintentional behaviours, rather than by the enhancement of creative thinking. These results were mostly supported by Abraham et al.; however, in contrast these authors also found that individuals with lesions in the basal ganglia and frontopolar areas demonstrated *increased* performance in presence of semantic constraints when generating creative responses (2012). Drago et al. reported on a single visual artist with Lewy body dementia (LBD), where representational ratings for the pictures painted when LBD was present were lower than for the pictures painted before development of LBD (2006). All the artistic qualities measures gradually declined except *novelty*. De Souza et al. also included patients with Parkinson's disease (PD), but these demonstrated no different results with regards to the TTCT in relation to controls (2010). Canesi et al. suggested that any increased artistic-like production in patients with PD is not due to impulsivity or impulsive control disorders, but rather embody innate skills in a subset of predisposed patients with PD released by dopaminergic therapy (2012).

Other mental disorders

A few studies and mental illnesses do not fall into any of the categories reviewed above. For example, studies including prominent individuals (big-C) have often reported increased occurrence of other mental disorders. Ludwig's study of 1005 eminent individuals revealed that those active within the creative arts had an increased occurrence of anxiety disorders (1992, 1995). Post also suggested frequent presence of unusual personality traits in his study of 291 world-famous men (1994). Glover and Tramel investigated students aged 14–19 years without (n = 200) and with (n = 194) behavioural problems, and found that those having behavioural problems scored significantly higher on flexibility and originality, than did students with no behavioural problems (1976). Akinola and Mendes reported that social rejection was associated with greater artistic creativity, and that this was especially evident among those lower in the hormone dehydroepiandrosterone (DHEAS). The latter was mediated through an increase in negative emotions, implicating DHEAS as a sign of affective vulnerability (2008). However, Smith and Carlsson argued that anxiety did not facilitate creativity in *patients* with anxiety disorders, while the opposite was the case for healthy controls (1983). The authors concluded that the main limitation to creative functioning is low tolerance of the anxiety associated with creative efforts.

Suicide and suicide ideation has also been explored in relation to creativity. Mraz and Runco found that problem generation scores were significantly correlated (*fluency* positively, *flexibility* negatively) with suicide ideation (1994). Preti et al. examined suicide rates in a sample of 4564 eminent artists who died in the nineteenth and twentieth centuries (2001). Musicians as a group had lower suicide rates than literary and visual artists. Stack used official suicide statistics and reported that artists had a 125 per cent higher risk of suicide than non-artists (1996). In our nation-wide study, artists had a small increase in anxiety disorders, but not in committed suicides (Kyaga et al., 2012). However, as in many previous studies authors singled out having a significant increase in most psychiatric disorders as well as in committed suicide. In general these increases revealed no familial pattern. Results also suggested a positive association of overall creative professions with anorexia nervosa. A study not included in the review but often referred to as demonstrating a 'Syliva Plath effect' is a study by Kaufman suggesting that female poets are especially prone to developing mental illness (Kaufman, 2001).

McNeil's study (1971), previously discussed in Chapter 5, compared 43 adults adopted by non-biologically related families to 23 non-creative adoptees. Mental illness rates in the adoptees were positively correlated to creative abilities, as were mental illness rates of their biological parents, but mental illness rates among adoptive parents were independent of the adoptees' creative abilities.

Summary of findings in literature review

Psychotic and mood disorders

There is an apparent consistency in findings of studies on psychotic and mood disorders in relation to creativity. First, none of the studies included in the literature review have indicated increases in general creative abilities in patients with schizophrenia. We demonstrated a specific increase in artistic occupations in patients with schizophrenia (Kyaga et al., 2011), but we were unable to validate these findings in a larger sample (Kyaga et al., 2013).

Second, in contradistinction to studies on patients with schizophrenia, all included studies reviewed reported associations between varied aspects of creativity and subsyndromal psychotic symptoms (psychoticism and schizotypy). Two studies, however, argued that schizotypy was mainly associated with self-reported creative abilities (Miller and Tal, 2007; Schuldberg, 2005). Miller et al. proposed that the increase in verbal and drawing creativity for schizotypy was mainly due to a correlated increase in Big five personality trait openness to experience. However, other authors have commented that this interpretation is based on the assumption that the effect of openness to experience has to be excluded from that of schizotypy, while the data are equally consistent with a path model where openness to experience fully mediates the effect of schizotypy on creativity (schizotypy increases openness to experience, which in turn augments creativity) (Del Giudice et al., 2010). Consistent with the findings on subsyndromal symptoms being associated with creativity, studies also generally affirm an association for non-diagnosed relatives of patients. We reported an overall association for healthy relatives of patients with schizophrenia (and bipolar disorder) for creative professions on a total population level (Kyaga et al., 2013; Kyaga et al., 2011). The results of these studies suggest an underlying genetic explanation for the association of creativity and psychotic disorders.

Third, quite a few studies support that patients with bipolar disorder have increased creative abilities, a finding also present in their non-diagnosed relatives. Some studies also suggest a similar association for the affective temperament. Fourth, the association between unipolar depression (major depressive disorder) and creativity is more ambiguous. Studies investigating prominent individuals (big-C) have indicated an increased occurrence in depression. However, most studies investigating patients with major depressive disorder do not support increased creative abilities in these patients. Comparable negative findings are also reported in relatives to these patients.

Neurodevelopmental disorders

Far fewer studies have investigated a possible link between creativity and neurodevelopmental disorders than for psychotic and mood disorders. While distinguished researchers such as Michael Fitzgerald and Simon Baron-Cohen have noticeably argued for a relation between autism and exceptional achievements, mainly in terms of a greater aptitude for scientific accomplishments, the empirical support is considerably weaker (Baron-Cohen et al., 2009; Fitzgerald, 2004). Mostly, a few selected historical individuals, such as Ludwig Wittgenstein, are referenced in support for the hypothesis (Fitzgerald, 2004). Some empirical support has been provided in a few studies of non-diagnosed relatives of patients with autism (Baron-Cohen et al., 1998; Campbell and Wang, 2012). No study has shown that autism itself would be beneficial for creativity. Correspondingly in ADHD, where there have also been suggestions of increased creativity, empirical support is limited. Studies included in the review largely give no such support among children with ADHD, but some support is provided in a few studies of adults with ADHD and possibly among those with subclinical syndromes (Healey and Rucklidge, 2006; White and Shah, 2006, 2011). Our nation-wide study gives little support for an association of ADHD or autism with creative professions, albeit non-diagnosed siblings of patients with autism were overrepresented in overall creative professions (Kyaga et al., 2013). This increase was particularly pronounced in the subgroup of scientific occupations. However, both parents and offspring to patients in this study demonstrated no comparable overrepresentation in creative professions. The idea that children with learning disability disorders are superior to their peers in creative capacities is on the whole not supported empirically.

Substance use/abuse

Some conclusions can be drawn from the studies reviewed. First, acute alcohol intoxication seems to have a positive effect on creative thinking. Results support increased divergent thinking, but also a more positive evaluation of intoxicated individuals with regards to their own creativity. The latter might not be due to the pharmacological effects of alcohol, but rather that people apply more lenient standards evaluating their creativity when they believe to be intoxicated (Lang et al., 1984). Second, studies suggest that alcohol abuse in the long run is not advantageous for creative productivity. Third, there does not seem to be a familial pattern associating alcohol abuse with creativity. Finally, the acute effects of other drugs on creative performance lack research. Long term use of drugs is probable not advantageous for creativity.

Neurological disorders

Investigations of creativity in relation to neurological disorders can be seen as a part of the recent surge of studies exploring the neural underpinnings of the creative process. In essence, however, there is little empirical support that any neurological disorder might enable a sustained increase in creativity.

Other mental disorders

Of the studies on creativity and mental illnesses that do not fall into any of the categories above, some propose an increased occurrence of anxiety disorders, behavioural problems, and affective vulnerability. Our nation-wide study suggested a small increase of anxiety disorders in artistic occupations (Kyaga et al., 2013). On the other hand, Smith and Carlsson argued that the main hindrance to creative functioning is low tolerance to the anxiety accompanying creative efforts (1983).

There are conflicting results regarding suicide and creativity. Our study did not provide any support for an increase of suicide in overall creative professions. However, as in many previous studies authors singled out having a significant increase in most psychiatric disorders as well as in suicide. Overall, these increases revealed no familial pattern.

Critique of studies

The results presented in the literature review gives a rather unanimous support for different aspects of creativity being associated with specific psychiatric syndromes, i.e., bipolar disorder, and subclinical features within the psychotic and affective domain manifested in healthy individuals. However, some of these studies have attracted serious methodological concerns. Some authors are defiant to the idea of mental illness having anything to do with creativity, and hold that there still is no (Rothenberg, 1995, 2001; Schlesinger, 2009, 2012, 2014) or very weak empirical support for any association (Sawyer, 2012a, 2012b).

The insanity hoax

The most vocal of those questioning the mad genius link is the psychologist Judith Schlesinger, who in her in 2012 book *The Insanity Hoax* contends that 'The mad genius is a beloved cultural artifact, a popular spectacle, and a favorite playing-field leveler... There is simply no good reason to believe that exceptionally creative people are more afflicted with psychopathology than anyone else' (p. 171). Her main criticism is that the authors of studies supporting the alleged association both selected study subjects and in general made the diagnoses themselves without support of recognized diagnostic manuals. This would make the results both open to bias and lead to difficulties in generalization.

Schlesinger argues that the myth about creativity and psychopathology is imminent in our society. Even as young children, we are exposed: 'Not only is this indoctrination broad, but it starts early. Magic Tree House is a popular children's series that introduces Leonardo da Vinci in Book #38, *Monday with a Mad Genius*' (p. 5). 'By now, everyone knows that there's a "fine line between genius and madness" – if only because they hear it so often. But is there any scientific truth to it? *Nope*' (p. 7).

'Let me be clear: I am not saying there are *no* creative people with genuine psychological problems, whether their diagnosis is bipolar disorder or anything else. Of course there are – just as there are erratic and unhappy lawyers and librarians, teachers and telemarketers. The distortion occurs when the great creatives are said to be more susceptible to this suffering than other groups, and studies are massaged to "prove" it' (p. 12). Schlesinger also suggests that there are often private reasons for professionals holding certain theories, 'One last observation on the link between professionals and their theories. I have noticed that most of the experts who regularly pass along the mad genius doctrine – and with so little attention to its flaws – are not psychotherapists. With doctorates in social or educational psychology, and careers spent in academic rather than clinical settings, they miss out on the regular, intimate revelations of living creative people' (p. 35).

Schlesinger provides a broad overview of the history of the genius (see also Chapter 2 in this book), and then pursues some of the major works on the mad genius link completed during the turn of the twentieth century, such as Lombroso and Galton (Galton, 1869; Lombroso, 1891), while also discussing J.F. Nisbet and Sigmund Freud (Schlesinger, 2012). She concludes with some references to Ellis, Lange-Eichbaum, and Juda (see Chapter 3) (Ellis, 1904; Juda, 1949; Lange-Eichbaum, 1928; Lange-Eichbaum and Paul, 1931), stressing their findings in contradiction to the ideas of Lombroso and others as genius inevitably linked to degeneration.

The main bulk of Schlesinger's criticism is heavily focused at only three studies; albeit studies that are often referred to as landmark studies of contemporary investigators affirming the mad genius link. These are Andreasen's study on creative writers at the Iowa writer's workshop (1987), Jamison's study of British artists and authors (1989), and Ludwig's compilation of just over a thousand prominent individuals (1992, 1995). The results of these studies were reviewed earlier in this chapter.

Schlesinger's critique of Andreasen's study revolves around four main problems (Schlesinger, 2009). The *first* is that Andreasen herself made all the diagnoses fully aware of whom she was meeting. An information bias (see below) might thus have been introduced leading to misclassification due to the information on subjects' profession not having been blinded to Andreasen (Ghaemi, 2009). This may also have been augmented by the fact that Andreasen used a self-developed instrument to aid diagnostics. While the latter is true, Schlesinger fails to acknowledge that most of the world uses the ICD to make diagnoses, which relies on prototypical diagnoses and clinical judgement rather than structured manuals (World Health Organization, 1967, 1977, 2004). Still, given that Andreasen was less restricted by structured manuals for diagnosing, this may have worsened potential misclassification further. Schlesinger's *second* critique is that there may have been a selection bias (see below), in that writers applying for the Iowa writer's workshop may have done so suffering setbacks and in order to recover from burnout (Schlesinger, 2009). This would make these writers more susceptible to psychiatric disorder than average writers. In addition the group of writers at Iowa was mainly male (27 of 30) with a mean age of 37, which would make the results only generalizable to this group. Finally, Andreasen's study of relatives to writers resulted from secondary sources; she did not meet them in person. While these are all legitimate concerns, they are not new. Albert Rothenberg had already raised these counterarguments ten years earlier (1995, 2001). Contrary to Schlesinger, Rothenberg also contributed with interesting empirical data contradicting a link between creativity and psychopathology (Rothenberg, 1983). In 1983 he published a study in which he assessed a type of creative cognition, which he termed janusian thinking (opposite response). Timed word association tests were administered to 12 creative scientists who were Nobel laureates, 18 hospitalized patients, and 113 college students divided as controls into high and low creative groups. The individually administered word association test involved the verbal presentation of 100 words. The subject was then instructed merely to give the first word that came to mind after each word presentation. The procedure allowed both a score for speed, but also a scoring category of verbal opposites, for example, sour as a response to sweet, or white as a response to black. A very rapid opposite response was suggested to indicate the janusian process of creative cognition. Results found that Nobel laureates gave the highest proportion of opposite responses at the fastest rate of all groups, whereas patients gave the lowest proportion of opposite responses, and at the slowest rate. However, an important aspect of the study was that Nobel laureates only included *scientists* (physics ($n = 5$), chemistry ($n = 2$), and medicine and physiology ($n = 5$)), and they were all males with ages ranging from 44 to 73 years. With regards to the patients included, these were hospitalized with a mixed range of diagnoses (schizophrenia ($n = 2$), borderline personality disorder ($n = 9$), brief reactive psychosis ($n = 1$), major depressive disorder ($n = 2$), anorexia nervosa ($n = 1$), opioid abuse ($n = 1$), alcohol dependence ($n = 1$), narcissistic personality disorder ($n = 1$). There were four men and 14 women among patients, and their ages ranged from 19 to 40 years. Five patients were receiving psychotropic medication and 13 were not. This group was simply lumped together as 'patients'. The included students divided into a high creative (n = 63) and a low creative (n = 50) student group were Yale University undergraduates. Being high creative or low creative was defined on the basis of an assessment of documented creative achievements in the arts and sciences and the strength of their creative interests. All students were male and ranged in age from 16 to 22 years. No distinction was reported with regards to artistic or scientific achievements or interests. The analyses did not account for differences in sex, age, domain of creativity in the different groups, or type of diagnosis in the patient group. Given this, Rothenberg's criticism of Andreasen for matching her controls on age, education, and sex but not on variables of occupation, intelligence, or achievements is slightly incoherent (Rothenberg, 1995).

Thus, considering that Rothenberg's study is often used as argument against the results of Andreasen's study, the critique does not seem fair. True, Andreasen did not use an acknowledged diagnostic manual, but then again Rothenberg did not even care about what diagnoses his patient group had. These were simply lumped together, and while there might have been selection bias in Andreasen's study from a selected group of authors seeking the Iowa writers' workshop, Rothenberg only included *inpatient*-treated patients. Clearly being eligible for inpatient treatment suggests that one might have problems with everyday activities. To find that this group was less able to provide rapid and opposite responses is maybe not so surprising. Finally, the critique of Andreasen using secondary sources for her investigation of relatives of writers may be legitimate, but then again Rothenberg did not even bother to investigate relatives of patients at all. These counterarguments are not to say that Rothenberg's study is without merit or that Andresen's study is without limitations. Quite the opposite, but the strengths and weaknesses of individual studies need to be assessed also in relation to what previous scientific literature was present upon publication. As will be evident below, Schlesinger's critique seems to be oddly aimed on proving her point by single-mindedly focusing on studies published more than 20 years ago (Schlesinger, 2009, 2012, 2014). To this end she also criticizes the findings of Jamison in her study of award-winning British artists and authors, published the same year as Andreasen's study (Jamison, 1989).

Schlesinger's critique of Jamison's work echoes those concerns stated for Andreasen's study (2009, 2012); Jamison did the interviews alone, 'like Andreasen's participants, they were all male and white, which once again precludes the fair application of results outside that gender, race, and age group, as well as non-award winners' (2012, p. 97). Schlesinger rightly points out that Jamison's study did not include a control group; however, prevalence rates in the general population are known and may be used as a reference (American Psychiatric Association and American Psychiatric Association. DSM-5 Task Force, 2013), although this prohibits the use of statistical hypothesis testing as Schlesinger also points out (Schlesinger, 2012). Overall, the critique delivered is more or less identical to that provided by Rothenberg some years earlier (Rothenberg, 1995). Schlesinger is also highly sceptical of Jamison's book *Touched with Fire: Manic-Depressive Illness and the Artistic Temperament*, in which Jamison aims to make a literary, biographical, and scientific association between the artistic and the manic-depressive temperaments (1996). Schlesinger disbelievingly refers to the book as the 'bible of the mad genius movement' (Schlesinger, 2012, p. 101).

Schlesinger's final rebuke concerns Ludwig's compilation of more than a thousand individuals, whose biographies had been reviewed in the *New York Times* book review from 1960 to 1990 (1992, 1995). The book, Schlesinger tells, is like 'Time-traveling back to Lombroso and the phrenologists' (2012, p. 106). Considering that Ludwig himself asserts that the results of his study demonstrate that mental illness is not essential for artistic success, Schlesinger's main concern seems to be that people don't read the contents of the book, but only the title: 'So why is this book considered proof that it is? The most obvious reason is that, once again, nobody's read it. In this case, the title seems to supply the answer by itself, since "the price of greatness" confirms that genius is psychologically inexpensive, while "resolving the creativity and madness controversy" suggests that the jury is in, sentence has been pronounced, and we can all go home' (2012, p. 106).

With the exception of some personal anecdotes from a debate held in the *British Journal of Psychiatry* in 2004 (Schlesinger, 2004; Wills, 2003), and a lash at historiometry in general and Dean Simonton in particular (Schlesinger, 2012, p. 126), the above concludes Schlesinger's critique. There is really no substantial new critique that has not already been commented by Rothenberg (Rothenberg, 1995). Rothenberg also quotes Juda and Ellis somewhat selectively in defending his point of view (Rothenberg, 2001), which also Keith Sawyer, a prominent creativity scholar, has adhered to more recently (Sawyer, 2012a, 2012b). For example, in his recent textbook on creativity Sawyer refers to Ellis saying that he 'found that only 4.2% had suffered from mental illness, 8% from melancholia, and 5% from personality disorder. These numbers weren't much higher than the general population, so he concluded that there was no relationship between genius and mental illness' (p. 166) (Sawyer, 2012b). This quote is similar to Rothenberg (Rothenberg, 2001), who claims that 'Ellis ... studied the biographies of 1,020 eminent persons listed in the *British Dictionary of National Biography* and diagnosed the following: 4.2% insane, 8% melancholic, 5% with traits suggestive of a personality disorder. No bipolar or manic-depressive illness was diagnosed in this early account and behaviour suggestive of that condition was described'. The reader is clearly given the impression that Ellis opposed the idea of an association between creativity and psychopathology. Yet, what Ellis actually wrote was, 'we find that the ascertainable number of cases of insanity is 44, so that the incidence of insanity among our 1,030 eminent persons is 4.2 per cent. It is perhaps a high proportion. I do not know the number of cases among persons of the educated classes living to a high average age in which it can be said that insanity has occurred at least once during life ... The association of genius with insanity is not, I believe, without significance, but in face of the fact that its occurrence is only demonstrable in less than 5 per cent cases, we must put out of court any theory as to genius being a form of insanity' (Ellis, 1904, p. 191). Similarly with regards to Juda's study, Rothenberg writes 'Juda ... investigated, primarily through psychiatric interviews, 294 German artists and scientists. She however, reported an incidence of only 1.3% manic-depressive psychosis and, for her overall results, concluded the following: "There is no definite relationship between highest mental capacity and psychic health or illness, and no evidence to support the assumption that the genesis of highest intellectual ability depends on psychic abnormalities"' (Rothenberg, 2001). Similarly, Sawyer quotes Juda writing, 'These numbers are only slightly higher than in the general population, and Juda concluded, "There is no definite relationship..."' (Sawyer, 2012b, p. 166). Again the reader is led to believe that Juda's view and results refuted an association between creativity and psychopathology (Juda, 1949). But in fact, Rothenberg's referral to the 294 individuals included demonstrated that 2.7 per cent of the artists suffered schizophrenia, while this was present among 0.85 per cent in the general population (Juda, 1949). There was also a high incidence of less severe psychopathology affecting in total a third of artists, for which Juda suggested that 'The very genesis of the complicated psychic pattern of artists *favours* the concomitant formation of gene combinations which result in a psychopathic disposition. It may be argued that certain qualities such as hypersensitivity, rapidly changing emotions, and even depressive inner experiences had, in some instances, a stimulating effect on the activation of creative ideas'. Further, Juda found that brothers and sisters to artists more often exhibited psychopathology than the general population: 'The number of schizophrenics corresponds to the general population, whereas the manic-depressives are twice as frequent as in the average population and the total figure for endogenous insanity is definitely higher than in average people.' With regards to children of artists: 'The incidence of endogenous psychoses was 4.1% and definitely increased as compared with 2% of the average population.' Additional investigation of 246 adult offspring to artists demonstrated that 21.5% had a cyclothymic constitution and 13.4% schizothymic constitution, suggesting 'a predominance of the cyclothymic temper in the families of the highly gifted artists'.

Among scientists, Juda found that results were reversed to those in artists, with an absence of schizophrenia, but 3.9 per cent (7 individuals of 181) suffering 'manic-depressive insanity' compared to 0.4 per cent in the average population. Juda remarks: 'In manic-depressive psychosis ... we find suppression of creative activity during the attack but revival of the original intellectual power during intermission... This raises the question of a certain correlation between the cyclothymic constitution and the highest mental ability.' With regards to siblings and children of scientists, they exhibited similar rates of psychopathology as did the relatives of artists.

Finally in the cohort that Rothenberg actually refers to, including only 115 artists and scientists of 'higher above-average intellect' but not considered geniuses, results demonstrated that this group suffered both schizophrenia (1.3 per cent) and 'manic-depressive psychosis' (1.3 per cent). Juda concluded, 'The evaluation of these findings shows that endogenous psychoses were less frequent than in the geniuses but more frequent than in the average population. The number of psychopaths appears to be very high and close to the figures found in the geniuses group.'

In a comment to the publication of our nation-wide study demonstrating an association between creative professions and psychopathology (Kyaga et al., 2013), Sawyer contends 'There is no link between creativity and mental illness. Creative people are not more likely to be diagnosed with mental illness, and mentally ill people are not more likely to be creative than normal people. Multiple studies, going back over a century, have consistently found the same proportion of mental illness in creative people as we find in the general population' (Sawyer, 2012a). He then refers to the above studies by Ellis (Ellis, 1904), Juda (Juda, 1949), and two studies by Goertzel and Goertzel (Goertzel, 1965), and Post (Post, 1994). While the book by Goertzel and Goertzel displays considerably less scientific rigour than the study by Juda (no control group or other base line), results are categorized as 'opionative parents', 'failure prone fathers', 'domineering mothers', 'smothering mothers', etc. for which no comparisons are made with regards to subgroups or average population nor with each other (Gowan, 1963). Results from the study by Post are again reported selectively. Sawyer writes, 'In 1994, Felix Post published a study of 291 biographies of famous men. None of these geniuses met the criteria for any DSM-III psychiatric diagnosis' (Sawyer, 2012b). The reader is clearly given the impression that Post reported no association for creativity and psychopathology, whereas the opposite is true. Post writes: 'Surprisingly, the biographies offered sufficient information to allow DSM-III-R diagnoses to be made with some confidence. Difficulties only arose in two areas: in the case of major depressive episodes (296.2 x or 3 x) this diagnosis requires, apart from the presence of either depressed mood or markedly diminished interest or pleasure, the presence of at least three of seven additional symptoms. Information on these was incomplete in most biographies. Provided the affective disorder had been present continuously for at least two weeks, depressive disorder not otherwise specified (311.00) was diagnosed when fewer than three additional criteria had been reported by the biographer.' (Post, 1994). Given this approach, Post reported increased rates of 'alcoholism (strikingly in writers, artists, and composers, less so in politicians and intellectuals, not at all in scientists)' and 'depressions (but markedly only in novelists and playwrights)' compared to the general population; however, no increased amount of psychoses in his sample compared to the general population. In all, using Post's findings to argue that there is no association between creativity and psychopathology seems, to borrow Schlesinger's words, quite frankly to 'massage' his data. This is not to say Post's study had no limitations, it clearly did and Post also admitted to some of them freely: 'I did not even try to entice another psychiatrist to share with me some ten years' work entailed in the careful reading of more than 350 biographies and the analysis of resulting data in an attempt to produce a definitive statement on the prevalence of psychic abnormalities and their distribution among a variety of men who had gained universal renown for their originating achievements.'

Sawyer concludes: 'Despite almost a century of work attempting to connect creativity and mental illness, evidence in support of a connection has been remarkably difficult to find. ...The consensus of all major creativity researchers today is that there's no link between mental illness and creativity' (Sawyer, 2012a). Yet, prominent scholars as George Becker rather claim the opposite; there is an emerging consensus that views the association between creativity and psychopathology as genuine and pervasive (Becker, 2014).

It may be questioned though if Schlesinger will ever consider an association between creativity and psychopathology being real. In 2009, she writes that the opportunity to answer this question was lost given that 'neither the National Institute of Mental Health nor the National Depressive and Manic-Depressive Association keeps statistics on the rate of mental illness by occupation' (Schlesinger, 2009), and that 'In 1999, the National Institute of Mental Health might have done it, when it launched its Systematic Treatment Enhancement Program for Bipolar Disorder (STEP-BD) study'. The STEP-BD was 'a $22 million, nationwide, longitudinal effort to find the most effective treatments for bipolar disorder ("$22 million," 2001). Completed in 2005, STEP-BD ultimately involved 19 research sites and an unprecedented pool of 4,361 bipolar participants. The largest study of its kind ever conducted, it was the perfect opportunity to finally answer the ancient question about creative madness – except that nobody asked it' (Schlesinger, 2009). Schlesinger concludes thus: 'There is still no clear, convincing, scientific proof that artists do, in fact, suffer more psychological problems than any other vocational group – and probably little chance of obtaining any.' However, in 2011 we demonstrated exactly this (Kyaga et al., 2011). Our study included 301457 patients on a nationwide basis diagnosed with schizophrenia, bipolar disorder, or unipolar depression, and results showed that patients with bipolar disorder more often reported having artistic and scientific occupations than healthy controls from the general population. Results also demonstrated that this increase was present among first-degree healthy relatives of patients with schizophrenia or bipolar disorder. Further, we expanded our cohort two years later and again demonstrated similar findings (Kyaga et al., 2013). Nevertheless, Schlesinger today still contends that there is no hard proof that highly creative people are more susceptible to mental disorder than anybody else (Schlesinger, 2014). While I applaud sound scepticism and adhere to the limitations pointed out in the studies by Andreasen, Jamison and Ludwig, Schlesinger rather gives the impression of being firm on proving her point than listening to what empirical results actually reveal.

In that sense, it is fitting that Schlesinger, with few exceptions, refrains from quoting any of the studies published the last 20 years on creativity and psychopathology (Schlesinger, 2009, 2012, 2014). As reviewed previously in this chapter, many of these studies complement findings provided by earlier studies with regards to such limitations as lack of controls, standardized diagnostics, and number of included subjects.

A summary of current knowledge

Thys et al. recently systematically reviewed studies on the association between creativity and psychopathology (2014a, 2014b), in which they concluded that 83 of a total of 111 included studies had been published after 1990. A hierarchy of included studies based on their design and according to 'hierarchy of research evidence in biomedical etiological research' was adopted, in which population studies (5 studies) were followed by comparative studies (48 studies), which in turn was followed by noncomparative studies (47 studies), and finally historical studies (11 studies). Thus, Andreasen's study would classify as a comparative study (1987), Jamison's study as a noncomparative study (1989), and Ludwig's as a historical study (1995). To a large extent studies included by Thys et al. are the same as those previously reviewed in this chapter. The benefit of the systematic approach is to give a more complete overview than casual references to sporadically chosen studies in the field, or sweeping referrals to 'The consensus of all major creativity researchers today...' (Sawyer, 2012a).

A broad overview of results in the studies included by Thys et al. provide the following, 75 of the studies (67.6 per cent) support a positive association between creativity and psychopathology, 25 (22.5 per cent) no association and 11 (9.9 per cent) a negative association. Thys et al. suggests that these relationships are to be considered carefully, as they mostly report a positive, absent or negative association with one or only a few psychiatric disorders. This is not least evident in studies investigating schizotypy, where psychiatric disorders were generally not investigated. A negative finding or findings not supporting any association thus only refers to schizotypy and not any psychiatric disorders or other subsyndromal traits, while a positive finding similarly only refers to schizotypy. The only study to assess a broad category of different psychiatric disorders with a substantial number of patients included is our study on ~1.2 million patients estimating occurrence of creative professions (artistic and scientific) in comparison to healthy controls from the general population (Kyaga et al., 2013). The disorder and subsyndromal features most frequently correlated with creativity is bipolar disorder and schizotypy (Thys et al., 2014b). Mood disorders and associated traits as a whole (bipolar disorder, cyclothymia, mania and depression) were positively correlated with creativity in 38 studies and psychosis as a whole (schizophrenia, schizotypy and psychoticism) in 33 studies. Thys et al. suggests that four studies report positive findings with regards to schizophrenia; however, one of these assessed artistic occupations in relation to *psychotic affective syndrome* (Muntaner et al., 1991), two were the studies by us (Kyaga et al., 2013; Kyaga et al., 2011), in which we found a small but significant increase of artistic occupations in the comparable smaller cohort that we were later unable to replicate in a larger cohort. Thus, only one study demonstrated an increased tendency for nonparanoid schizophrenics (n = 10) to outperform healthy controls (n = 10) on the Alternate uses test measuring divergent thinking; however, this was not statistically significant (p<.10) (Keefe and Magaro, 1980). Thus, no study gave good support for an association of schizophrenia disorder and creativity being positively correlated, while seven studies found a negative association between schizophrenia and creativity (Thys et al., 2014b). Thys et al. also confirmed that an association to other psychiatric disorders (e.g., personality disorders, anxiety, autism) is supported only in a small numbers of studies (for an overview see studies previously reviewed in this chapter), but has also seldom been investigated. Nine studies found that first-degree relatives of psychiatric patients were overrepresented in creative occupations, while one study focusing on relatives of alcoholics found a negative association (Noble et al., 1993).

The above gives an indication of where the field stands today with regards to the empirical support for an association between creativity and psychopathology. However, the results poignantly put by Thys et al. needs to be cautiously interpreted, given that many display inherent limitations (2014b). Further, Thys et al. also reported that of 111 creativity assessment tools and criteria used in the included studies, 74 were used in only one research article or by only one author.

Levels of evidence

Nassir Ghaemi, an international expert on bipolar disorder, has suggested that it is important to view results gathered from studies using various study designs as different levels of evidence rather than evidence or not (2009; Howick et al., 2011; La Caze, 2009). He provides a nice and accessible framework for interpreting the strengths of evidence gathered by different study designs with focus on treatment studies. This framework, consisting of both an evaluation of study design as well as of three fundamental features, i.e., confounding, chance and causation, is however also useful when considering studies on the association between creativity and psychopathology. In accordance with general guidelines for evidence-based medicine regarding study design, at the lowest level of evidence Ghaemi places case reports and expert opinions (level V). At level IV, are small observational studies where participants were not randomized and there is no control population, such as Jamison's study

(1989), whereas level III are larger observational studies. These are divided into medium-sized nonrandomized uncontrolled studies (level IIIc), large nonrandomized uncontrolled studies (level IIIb), such as Ludwig's study (Ludwig, 1995), and finally nonrandomized, controlled studies (level IIIa), such as Andreasen's study (1987). Level II and I are reserved for randomized trials, which with the exception of studies investigating the acute effects of substances on creative performance are generally not an option for investigating creativity and psychopathology (Lang et al., 1984; Lowe, 1994).

However, apart from recognizing these general rules in affirming weight to the findings of different studies according to their design, there are some fundamental aspects of individual studies that also need to be acknowledged. Ghaemi suggests that these may best be framed by the three Cs: confounding (i.e., systematic errors), chance and causation (Abramson et al., 2001).

Confounding (systematic errors)

The type of errors sorted under 'confounding' is generally referred to as bias or *systematic errors* (Rothman, 2012). Systematic errors denote a tendency to make the same mistake over and over again in a study. There are three types of systematic errors: selection bias, information bias and confounding.

Selection bias

Selection bias is the consequence when study subjects are selected as a result of an unknown variable associated with both the exposure and outcome investigated. For example, it was suggested that those attending the Iowa writer's workshop in Andreasen's study attended this workshop after suffering setbacks and burnout, which would make them suffer psychiatric disorders more than writers in general (Andreasen, 1987; Rothenberg, 1995, 2001; Schlesinger, 2009, 2012). Selection bias is also a major problem in most studies where prominent individuals were selected without any clear strategy (Lombroso, 1891; Rothenberg, 1983).

Information bias

Information bias refers to bias arising from measurement error (Rothman, 2012). This may lead to misclassifications of outcome and exposure resulting in false associations (type I error) or false negatives (type II error). Misclassification that is similar (non-differential) across groups (exposures, outcomes, and covariates) results in a diluted effect, while differential misclassification results in an overestimation or underestimation of effect. A common reason for information bias is *recall bias*. Information bias is therefore generally reduced in prospective designs. Importantly, studies that are *blinded* to the investigator (and if possible also to the investigated) tend to restrict information bias.

Misclassification in studies investigating creativity and psychopathology may arise from either a lack of information, such as in Post's study (Post, 1994), but could also be due to unclear definitions of diagnosis, for example, lack of structured manuals for diagnosis (Andreasen, 1987), or by assessors being unskilled in using existing instruments. Given that the use of structured manuals for diagnosis was not broadly implemented before the 1980s, most studies published before 1980 can be suspected to be based on clinical evaluations rather than strict criteria. However, for example Dykes and Mcghie utilized diagnoses made independently by two different psychiatrists to strengthen validity (1976). In addition, the varying definitions of creativity also constitute potential information bias (Thys et al., 2014a). Thys et al. conclude that the plethora of different instruments compromises the comparability, the generalizability and therefore the value of research. Some instruments are suggested to be too subjective, such as expert judgement by only one person (Sitton and Hughes, 1995), and self-rating of creativity (Barbato et al., 2007; Batey and Furnham, 2008; Brand et al., 2011; Ludwig, 1994; Schou, 1979), while many instruments have also never been validated (Thys et al., 2014a). This is truly a waste of resources, given that established instruments for most presently defined aspects of creativity are around (see Chapter 4).

Confounding

A confounder is a variable associated with both exposure and outcome resulting in a spurious association. Experimental studies may randomize participants in order to handle possible confounding; however, observational studies do not have that alternative. Therefore, matching or stratifying controls according to known variables is often used to deal with possible confounding. In regression models there is also the option of adjusting for a possible confounder. Studies investigating creativity and psychopathology may display a number of confounders; one possibility is that any associations found between, for example, artists and psychiatric disorders may reflect social drift rather than creativity (Kyaga et al., 2013; Kyaga et al., 2011). It is also important to consider aspects, such as age, gender, socioeconomic factors, and IQ.

Chance

Random errors are errors caused by chance. If observational data are appropriately analysed with care taken to systematic errors, and there still seems to be an association, then results need to be assessed for being chance findings. In general, larger samples result in the precision of findings increasing, which means that estimates are less susceptible to chance. The convention is that a p-value of less than 0.05 is considered unlikely to be erroneous.

Thus, Lauronen et al. reviewed studies on creativity and psychopathology including over 100 individuals in 2004 and concluded that of the 13 included studies having valid, reliable measures of mental disorders, all but one supported an association (2004). Some of the included studies, however, were uncontrolled (i.e., level IIIc and IIIb), and therefore were not eligible for assessing standard p-values.

Causation

If potential bias has been reasonably handled, chance has been minimized, but there is still the problem of inferring causation. Causation is the whole point of research. It is not a statistical question, but rather a philosophical problem (Ghaemi, 2009).

Causality may seem unpretentious at first: the sun rises every day, and we therefore infer that the sun causes the day. It is simply reasonable to assume that the sun causes the day, but in fact it is quite possible that someday the sun will not rise, and we will still have a new day. This is what is concluded in Hume's law, referring to the Scottish philosopher David Hume (1711–76). To put it in another way, observations in the real world cannot prove that one thing causes another, i.e., *induction* fails. Hume's arguments made many philosophers search for *deduction* of causality, as in mathematical proofs.

But, how can you prove causation when you are dealing with human beings? If it was possible to consider animal studies on the putative association between creativity and psychopathology, then one could, for example, control for *genetics* by breeding for specific genetic types or control the *environment* in a laboratory also so that animals can be studied on the basis that they only differ on the one variable investigated. But such experiments are neither possible nor ethical with humans.

Two fundamental facts have been the reason for much unnecessary scientific conflict over the years: the recognition that induction can be faulty and the mistaken notion that causation has to imply the cause (2009). Ghaemi gives a nice illustration of this in describing the discussions on the potential health risks of tobacco ignited in the 1950s (Ghaemi, 2009). Before the 1950s, the US tobacco industry was booming, and the public had little insight into the effects of tobacco on their health. However, in 1950 A. Bradford Hill and his associate Richard Doll investigated 709 patients with lung cancer at 20 London hospitals, and matched these patients by age and gender to 709 patients without lung cancer. They demonstrated an association between reported smoking and lung cancer. It was not definitive, but it was stronger than what would have been expected by chance. The main question was, could there be other factors causing the association, i.e., systematic errors? Hill and Doll held that other causes were unlikely. But there were many limitations in their claim; no animal studies had found specific carcinogens in cigarette smoke and, argued the tobacco industry, the main source of data was patient recall about historical smoking habits known to be faulty, and finally, said the industry, other conceivable causes existed, such as environmental pollution, which had increased in the last decades and which also nicely correlated with findings of lung cancer being present more in cities than in rural areas.

Hill's list

Hill was revolutionary in bringing randomization to clinical medical research by conducting the first randomized clinical trial (RCT) in 1948 on streptomycin for pneumonia. Yet, in addition to implementing RCTs in clinical research Hill also recognized that much of medicine was not open for RCTs and, therefore, he suggested methods to infer causation also in observational settings. Thus, although it is convention to stress that an association does not necessarily imply causation, the question is: when does it? To this end, Hill suggested a list of nine important aspects: strength of the association, consistency of the observation, specificity of the relationship, temporal association, biologic gradient (dose–response effect), plausibility, coherence with other evidence, experiment, and analogy (Hill, 1965).

Strength of the association   Hill argued that a large effect can be seen as strong evidence of causation. Other guidelines have stressed strength of associations as important and suggested that weak associations, for example, relative risks and odds ratios of less than 2, be discounted (Grimes and Schulz, 2012). It may be tempting to assume that strong associations are more probable to be causal than weak ones. However, it is not certain that every component cause has a strong association with the outcome that it produces. Ghaemi quotes Hill, 'We must not be too ready to dismiss a cause-and-effect hypothesis merely on the grounds that the observed association appears to be slight. There are many occasions in medicine when this is in truth so. Relatively few persons harbouring the meningococcus fall sick of meningococcal meningitis.' (Ghaemi, 2009, p. 74). A strong association makes causation probable, but a weak association does not, by itself, make causation unlikely. Most associations between creativity and psychopathology demonstrated in contemporary studies are weak, such as in our nation-wide studies on creative professions, where patients with bipolar disorder were roughly 35 per cent more likely to hold an artistic or scientific occupation compared to healthy controls from the general population (Kyaga et al., 2011). Kenneth Rothman, author of two widely used textbooks on epidemiologic methods (2012; Rothman et al., 2008), argues that if weak associations can be causal and strong associations can be noncausal, for example due to confounding, then the strength of association in itself cannot be considered a criterion for causality. Rather than simple checklists, Rothman argues for a process based on conjecture and refutation echoing Karl Popper (Popper, 2002). Thus, we need also to take into account other aspects in order to consider putative causation.

Consistency of the association   Findings need to be replicated. This is not least important when considering studies on potential genes underlying creativity, but also of major importance in view of the literature on creativity and psychopathology. Replication does not mean that the same study should necessarily be performed again, but rather that the research question needs to be addressed with different methods. Studies investigating creativity and psychopathology have addressed different aspects of creativity and, as was previously reviewed, using different study designs. Thys et al. found that of 121 studies investigating an association between creativity and psychopathology, most tapped into the creative person or the creative process, while some studies also addressed the creative product (2014a). As previously mentioned, it was found that of 111 studies, 75 (67.6 per cent) supported a positive association between creativity and psychopathology, 25 (22.5 per cent) no association, and 11 (9.9 per cent) a negative association (Thys et al., 2014b). Of the 111 studies, most investigated subsyndromal psychotic symptoms (n = 36), such as schizotypy, bipolar disorder (n = 18), and schizophrenia (n = 12).

Of the studies investigating subsyndromal psychotic syndromes including a control group (i.e., level IIIa; n = 14) (Thys et al., 2014b), 13 found a positive association, while one found no association (Rodrigue and Perkins, 2012). However, given that both schizotypy and creativity measurements are not necessarily categorical, studies reported as noncomparative also provide important evidence. Some of these have been reviewed above and include comparable large samples (Schuldberg, 2005).

Of 15 controlled studies investigating bipolar disorder, 14 suggest a positive association for creativity (Thys et al., 2014b). Some of these studies have been criticized on methodological grounds, for example Andreasen's study from 1987. However, more recent studies have addressed many of the suggested shortcomings of this study, such as in diagnostic validity (Kyaga et al., 2013; Kyaga et al., 2011; Rybakowski and Klonowska, 2011; Santosa et al., 2007; Simeonova et al., 2005; Soeiro-de-Souza et al., 2011; Srivastava et al., 2010), inclusion of controls (Kyaga et al., 2013; Kyaga et al., 2011; Rybakowski and Klonowska, 2011; Santosa et al., 2007; Simeonova et al., 2005; Soeiro-de-Souza et al., 2011; Soeiro-de-Souza et al., 2012; Srivastava et al., 2010), both genders and different ages (Kyaga et al., 2013; Kyaga et al., 2011; Rybakowski and Klonowska, 2011; Santosa et al., 2007; Simeonova et al., 2005; Soeiro-de-Souza et al., 2011; Soeiro-de-Souza et al., 2012; Srivastava et al., 2010). Finally, three of the studies were population studies including large samples, one including more than a million patients in total (68915 patients with bipolar disorder), as well as all of their first, second, and third degree relatives. Data on both diagnosis and creativity (creative professions) in two of the three population studies were collected prospectively and were on a total population level, thus not open for recall bias and minimizing selection bias (Kyaga et al., 2013; Kyaga et al., 2011).

As previously mentioned, with regards to schizophrenia, Thys et al. suggest that four studies provide support for a positive association to schizophrenia; however, one of these assessed artistic occupations in relation to *psychotic affective syndrome* (Muntaner et al., 1991), two were the studies by us (Kyaga et al., 2013; Kyaga et al., 2011), in which we were unable to replicate findings of a small but significant increase of artistic occupations. The last study reporting a trend for an increased tendency of nonparanoid schizophrenics (n = 10) to outperform healthy controls (n = 10) on the Alternate uses test measuring divergent thinking was not statistically significant (Keefe and Magaro, 1980). Thus, no study gave support for schizophrenia and creativity being positively correlated, while five controlled studies found a negative association (Thys et al., 2014b). On the other hand, our nation-wide study demonstrated an increased occurrence of creative professions (artistic and scientific) in healthy first-degree relatives of patients with schizophrenia in comparison with controls from the general population (Kyaga et al., 2011). These results were also found when we further increased the cohort (Kyaga et al., 2013).

Specificity of the association Studies on creativity and psychopathology do not find that all psychiatric disorders are associated with increased creative behaviour. For example, in our nation-wide study of creative professions, we included patients with schizophrenia, schizoaffective disorder, bipolar disorder, unipolar depression, anxiety disorders, alcohol abuse, drug abuse, autism, ADHD, anorexia nervosa, and completed suicide (Kyaga et al., 2013). This study only supported an association for patients with bipolar disorder. No other patient group demonstrated increased occurrence of overall creative professions. Further, bipolar disorder together with schizophrenia also exhibited clear increased occurrence of creative professions in healthy relatives, a finding not present in other disorders investigated. As mentioned above this, specificity is also supported in the literature overall.

Temporality Causes precede effects, which means that time is important. It was once suggested that the association between lung cancer and smoking could possibly be causative in either direction; persons with lung cancer could be more inclined to smoke in order to reduce pulmonary irritation caused by their cancers. However, Hill was able to show that most smokers started their habit when they were young, long before they developed lung cancer.

With creativity and psychopathology the question is more difficult. However, given that findings support increased creativity in subsyndromal symptoms, and healthy relatives of patients, and that both schizotypy and affective temperaments have been suggested to draw much on factors established on a genetic level (Evans et al., 2005; Keri, 2009; Lenzenweger, 2010), albeit integrating to some extent environmental factors and the individual person (e.g., her or his life story) (Stanghellini and Rosfort, 2010), we may conceive that traits precede creative expression. Nevertheless, this question needs to be further examined.

Biological gradient It has been suggested that the association between creativity and psychopathology follows an inverted-U relationship, in which the association with creativity peaks in first-degree relatives of those with a mental disorder, rather than in the patients themselves (Kyaga et al., 2011; Richards et al., 1988). Hence, in the absence of a debilitating illness, the relatives of those with schizophrenia or bipolar disorder might benefit from increased creativity.

Plausibility   Hill suggests that causative inference may be supported if it is biologically plausible (Ghaemi, 2009). This is a weak criterion since what is biologically plausible depends on current knowledge. Nevertheless, studies like Keri's proposing Neuregulin 1 (2009), a candidate gene, associated with both creative achievement and psychosis, as well as De Manzano and co-workers' finding of thalamic dopamine receptor D2 density in divergent thinking similar to psychosis (2010), may provide some biologic plausibility for an association between creativity and psychopathology.

Coherence   Coherence refers to the premise that suggested causative factors should not be in serious conflict with generally known facts. While the association between creativity and psychopathology has been the subject of a heated debate, it may still be conceived as coherent with what is generally known given that the limited biological data, clinical impressions, and layman's opinion does not clearly contradict the association.

Experiment   The *randomized experiment* where the exposure can be randomized to study participants is generally considered the gold standard to infer causation. However, for obvious practical and ethical reasons, the randomized experiment is not an option for investigating the association between creativity and psychopathology in humans. Thus, we are submitted to *observational studies* (level III) to investigate correlations, in which causal inference is restricted and unidentified factors may lead to biased results. For that reason *quasi-experimental designs* offer an interesting alternative. These may use family-based designs reducing genetic and environmental confounding, thereby providing indication of causality. Another option is to use *negative control analyses* to get an indication of the influence of confounding. In our nation-wide study on creative professions, we also investigated *accountants and auditors*, considered a less creative occupational group, as a negative control (Kyaga et al., 2013; Kyaga et al., 2011). This provided an opportunity to consider the effects of having an occupation in general – importantly, as a group accountants and auditors also demonstrated a similar IQ mean to that of the overall creative professions. In general, being an accountant or a relative to an accountant meant negative or no association to the psychopathologies investigated (Kyaga et al., 2013).

Analogy Hill also suggested that causation may be inferred through analogy. For example, since rubella is associated with pregnancy-related malformations, there may also be other viruses leading to similar malformations. Thus, we may infer that mania is associated with creativity given that there is good evidence of positive emotion being associated with state-dependent increased creativity (Baas et al., 2008). In fact, there is some support for mania being associated with creativity (Thys et al., 2014b), although there also seem to be individual differences (Soeiro-de-Souza et al., 2012).

To conclude, this chapter has reviewed and discussed contemporary studies on creativity and psychopathology, while addressing inherent limitations and support. The aim has been to provide a complete overview of studies performed, rather than to selectively consider certain studies. I have argued that there is reasonable support for an association between patients with bipolar disorder, subsyndromal psychotic features, and relatives to patients with bipolar disorder and schizophrenia with different aspects of creativity. These associations are specific, and most other psychiatric disorders have not been found to demonstrate similar associations, especially with regards to familiality (Kyaga et al., 2013).

7
Conclusion

This book is about the alleged association between creativity and mental illness. The aim has not been to establish a grand theory, but rather to provide a broad overview of current knowledge based on empirical observations, while also suggesting a framework of contemporary research literature related to this topic. Two chapters provided a brief historical perspective on both the varying view on creativity in general and the link to melancholic temperament, divine madness and eventually clinical insanity. It was suggested that the idea of the mad genius link is both old and comparably modern. While the Greeks suggested certain traits associated with eminence, the Romantics' emphasis on imagination over rationality served to provide intellectual independence. But soon genius was purported as a manifestation of an inescapable madness; an idea not least driven by the emerging medico-psychiatric field (Becker, 2014).

At the centre of this movement was Lombroso (1891), with his man of genius struck by insanity characterized by originality, but inevitably headed for degeneration; the innate traits of the genius emphasized by Galton (1869), both Lombroso and Galton were soon challenged by Lange-Eichbaum (1931), who maintained that the genius was only a genius owing to recognition by his or her fellow beings. But the final blow to Lombroso's ideas came with Juda's conclusion of most artists and scientists being mentally healthy (1949). Soon Guilford helped give birth to contemporary creativity research (1950), which left the confines of genius and instead included ordinary people's creativity in everyday life. Modern creativity research was established as an independent field of research, with an increasing number of psychometric tests assessing various aspects of creativity, practically abbreviated into the four Ps: personality, process, product and press (Rhodes, 1987).

Divergent thinking was placed at the centre of the creative *process*, facilitating the growth of theories not least on this process: associative theory, analogical thinking, and even problem solving, all theories stressing different aspects of the creative process. Some important facets of these theories, not least the inclusive Darwinian model of creativity by Simonton (1999a), heavily influenced by Campbell's blind variation and selective retention (1960), have been proposed in relation to the often surfaced idea of psychosis and bipolar disorder linked to creativity. The main question of this book has been to assess if there is empirical support for such an association.

Evidence

This question, still open for debate but with increasing evidence for support, was considered in the last chapter, where contemporary studies on creativity and psychopathology were reviewed and criticism discussed. I argue that, although with limitations, there is now reasonable support for an association between patients with bipolar disorder, subsyndromal psychotic features, and relatives to patients with bipolar disorder and schizophrenia with different aspects of creativity. This association may be explained within some of the theories alluded to above, as well as by burgeoning findings on the biology of creativity, such as in genetics and neuroscience. However, as for now, I am satisfied with answering the 'if', rather than the 'how'. Critics of the mad genius link may still not be content with present evidence, and ask for more. This is probably a good thing, given that the association between creativity and psychopathology is in the public's eye, and thus not only has bearing as a scholarly field, but also for psychiatric patients and for society as a whole.

Future

To this end, we may ask how to proceed? Gordon Claridge, a prominent psychologist with an interest in the field (2009), when commenting on our ~1.2 million patient nation-wide study on creative professions, said 'Looking to the future, it is perhaps now time to move beyond repeated studies of the more usual examples of "creative professions" – as reported here – and examine some different angles on the topic. Two examples I can quote from own recent work is showing similar connections in another creative group, adult comedians, and in individuals who reported having imaginary friends in childhood' (Claridge, 2012). Since then, Claridge has among other things published interesting findings on subsyndromal psychotic traits in comedians (Ando et al., 2014), while we have investigated bipolar disorder and superior leadership traits (Kyaga, 2014).

Purpose

What may the purpose be for investigating this question further? Of course the main reason is simply that we want to know more. But the association between creativity and psychopathology may also serve another important cause. Today, many do not want to live near or work with people who have, or have suffered, mental illness (Borelius et al., 2014). Workplaces generally lack effective support for those affected by mental disorder compared to those struck by somatic disease. When media talk about people who are mentally ill, four times out of ten the stories concern violence and crime. The time has truly come for mental disease to come out of that old closet of non-deserved shame. It is in this setting that research on creativity and psychopathology may provide a change; to give hope and optimism back to those struck by mental illness and their families.

References

Abraham, A., Beudt, S., Ott, D.V.M. and von Cramon, D.Y. (2012). Creative cognition and the brain: Dissociations between frontal, parietal-temporal and basal ganglia groups. *Brain Research, 1482*, 55–70. doi: DOI 10.1016/j.brainres.2012.09.007

Abraham, A., Windmann, S., McKenna, P. and Gunturkun, O. (2007). Creative thinking in schizophrenia: the role of executive dysfunction and symptom severity. *Cogn Neuropsychiatry, 12*(3), 235–58. doi: 10.1080/13546800601046714

Abraham, A., Windmann, S., Siefen, R., Daum, I. and Gunturkun, O. (2006). Creative thinking in adolescents with attention deficit hyperactivity disorder (ADHD). *Child Neuropsychol, 12*(2), 111–23. doi: 10.1080/09297040500320691

Abramson, J.H., Abramson, Z.H. and Abramson, J.H.S. m. i. c. m. (2001). *Making sense of data: A self-instruction manual on the interpretation of epidemiological data* (3rd ed.). Oxford: Oxford University Press.

Adams, F. (1849). *The Genuine Works of Hippocrates.* New York: W. Wood & Co.

ADHD-Awareness-Month (2014). Get the Facts ADHD Can Affect ANYONE. Retrieved 26 April, 2014, from http://www.adhdawarenessmonth.org/

Aggleton, J.P., Kentridge, R.W. and Good, J.M.M. (1994). Handedness and Musical Ability: A Study of Professional Orchestral Players, Composers & Choir Members. *Psychology of Music, 22*(2), 148–56. doi: 10.1177/0305735694222004

Ahn, C.W. (2006). *Advances in evolutionary algorithms: Theory, design and practice.* Berlin; New York: Springer.

Akinola, M. and Mendes, W.B. (2008). The dark side of creativity: biological vulnerability and negative emotions lead to greater artistic creativity. *Pers Soc Psychol Bull, 34*(12), 1677–86. doi: 0146167208323933 [pii] 10.1177/0146167208323933

Akiskal, H.S. and Akiskal, K.K. (2007). In search of Aristotle: Temperament, human nature, melancholia, creativity and eminence. *J Affect Disord, 100*(1–3), 1–6. doi: S0165–0327(07)00139–5 [pii] 10.1016/j.jad.2007.04.013

al-Issa, I. (1976). Creativity and overinclusion in chronic schizophrenia. *Psychol Rep, 38*(3 pt. 1), 979–82.

Amabile, T.M. (1982). Social-Psychology of Creativity – a Consensual Assessment Technique. *Journal of Personality and Social Psychology, 43*(5), 997–1013. doi: 10.1037/0022–3514.43.5.997

Amabile, T.M. (1996). *Creativity in context.* Boulder, Colo.: Westview Press.

Amabile, T.M. and Conti, R. (1999). Changes in the work environment for creativity during downsizing. *Academy of Management Journal, 42*(6), 630–40. doi: 10.2307/256984

Amabile, T.M. and Gryskiewicz, N.D. (1989). The creative environment scales: Work environment inventory. *Creativity Research Journal, 2*(4), 231–53. doi: 10.1080/10400418909534321

Amabile, T.M., Conti, R., Coon, H., Lazenby, J. and Herron, M. (1996). Assessing the work environment for creativity. *Academy of Management Journal, 39*(5), 1154–84. doi: 10.2307/256995

Amabile, T.M., Hill, K.G., Hennessey, B.A. and Tighe, E.M. (1994). The Work Preference Inventory – Assessing Intrinsic and Extrinsic Motivational Orientations. *Journal of Personality and Social Psychology, 66*(5), 950–67. doi: 10.1037/0022-3514.66.5.950

American Psychiatric Association & American Psychiatric Association. DSM-5 Task Force. (2013). *Diagnostic and statistical manual of mental disorders: DSM-5* (5th ed.). Washington, D.C.: American Psychiatric Association.

American Psychiatric Association. Task Force on Nomenclature and Statistics & American Psychiatric Association. Committee on Nomenclature and Statistics (1980). *Diagnostic and statistical manual of mental disorders* (3d ed.). Washington, D.C.: American Psychiatric Association.

Amin, F., Davidson, M. and Davis, K.L. (1992). Homovanillic acid measurement in clinical research: A review of methodology. *Schizophr Bull, 18*(1), 123–48.

Ando, V., Claridge, G. and Clark, K. (2014). Psychotic traits in comedians. *Br J Psychiatry*. doi: 10.1192/bjp.bp.113.134569

Andreasen, N.C. (1987). Creativity and mental illness: Prevalence rates in writers and their first-degree relatives. *Am J Psychiatry, 144*(10), 1288–92.

Andreasen, N.C. (2007). DSM and the death of phenomenology in america: an example of unintended consequences. *Schizophr Bull, 33*(1), 108–12. doi: sbl054 [pii] 10.1093/schbul/sbl054.

Andreasen, N.C. (2008). The relationship between creativity and mood disorders. *Dialogues Clin Neurosci, 10*(2), 251–5.

Andreasen, N.C. and Powers, P.S. (1974). Overinclusive thinking in mania and schizophrenia. *Br J Psychiatry, 125,* 452–6.

Andreasen, N.C. and Powers, P.S. (1975). Creativity and Psychosis - Examination of Conceptual Style. *Archives of General Psychiatry, 32*(1), 70–3.

Annett, M. and Kilshaw, D. (1982). Mathematical Ability and Lateral Asymmetry. *Cortex, 18*(4), 547–68.

Arden, R., Chavez, R.S., Grazioplene, R. and Jung, R.E. (2010). Neuroimaging creativity: A psychometric view. *Behav Brain Res, 214*(2), 143–16. doi: S0166-4328(10)00365-7 [pii] 10.1016/j.bbr.2010.05.015

Argulewicz, E.N., Mealor, D.J. and Richmond, B.O. (1979). Creative abilities of learning disabled children. *J Learn Disabil, 12*(1), 21–4.

Aristotle (1984). *The complete works of Aristotle: The revised Oxford translation* (J. Barnes, Trans.). Princeton, N.J.: Princeton University Press.

Asari, T., Konishi, S., Jimura, K., Chikazoe, J., Nakamura, N. and Miyashita, Y. (2008). Right temporopolar activation associated with unique perception. *Neuroimage, 41*(1), 145–52. doi: 10.1016/j.neuroimage.2008.01.059

Atchley, R.A., Keeney, M. and Burgess, C. (1999). Cerebral hemispheric mechanisms linking ambiguous word meaning retrieval and creativity. *Brain and Cognition, 40*(3), 479–99. doi: 10.1006/brcg.1999.1080

Aziz-Zadeh, L., Kaplan, J.T. and Iacoboni, M. (2009). 'Aha!': The neural correlates of verbal insight solutions. *Hum Brain Mapp, 30*(3), 908–16. doi: 10.1002/hbm.20554

Baas, M., De Dreu, C.K. and Nijstad, B.A. (2008). A meta-analysis of 25 years of mood-creativity research: Hedonic tone, activation, or regulatory focus? *Psychol Bull, 134*(6), 779–806. doi: 10.1037/a0012815

Bäck, T. (1996). *Evolutionary algorithms in theory and practice: Evolution strategies, evolutionary programming, genetic algorithms.* Oxford; New York: Oxford University Press.

Baer, J. (2003). The impact of the core knowledge curriculum on creativity. *Creativity Research Journal, 15*(2–3), 297–300. doi: 10.1207/S15326934crj152and3_20

Baer, J., Kaufman, J.C. and Gentile, C.A. (2004). Extension of the consensual assessment technique to nonparallel creative products. *Creativity Research Journal, 16*(1), 113–17. doi: DOI 10.1207/s15326934crj1601_11

Barbato, G., Piemontese, S. and Pastorello, G. (2007). Seasonal changes in mood and creative activity among eminent Italian writers. *Psychol Rep, 101*(3 Pt 1), 771–7.

Baron-Cohen, S., Bolton, P., Wheelwright, S., Scahill, V., Short, L., Mead, G. and Smith, A. (1998). Does Autism Occur More Often in Families of Physicists, Engineers and Mathematicians? *Autism, 2*, 296–301. doi: 10.1177/1362361398023008

Baron-Cohen, S., Ashwin, E., Ashwin, C., Tavassoli, T. and Chakrabarti, B. (2009). Talent in autism: hyper-systemizing, hyper-attention to detail and sensory hypersensitivity. *Philos Trans R Soc Lond B Biol Sci, 364*(1522), 1377–83. doi: 364/1522/1377 [pii]10.1098/rstb.2008.0337

Barron, F. (1970). Heritability of factors in creative thinking and esthetic judgment. *Acta Genet Med Gemellol (Roma), 19*(1), 294–98.

Barron, F. and Parisi, P. (1976). Twin resemblances in creativity and in esthetic and emotional expression. *Acta Genet Med Gemellol (Roma), 25*, 213–17.

Barron, F. and Harrington, D.M. (1981). Creativity, Intelligence and Personality. *Annual Review of Psychology, 32*, 439–76. doi: 10.1146/annurev.ps.32.020181.002255

Batey, M. and Furnham, A. (2008). The relationship between measures of creativity and schizotypy. *Personality and Individual Differences, 45*(8), 816–21. doi: 10.1016/j.paid.2008.08.014

Bechtereva, N.P., Korotkov, A.D., Pakhomov, S.V., Roudas, M.S., Starchenko, M.G. and Medvedev, S.V. (2004). PET study of brain maintenance of verbal creative activity. *Int J Psychophysiol, 53*(1), 11–20. doi: 10.1016/j.ijpsycho.2004.01.001

Bechtereva, N.P., Danko, S.G. and Medvedev, S.V. (2007). Current methodology and methods in psychophysiological studies of creative thinking. *Methods, 42*(1), 100–8. doi: 10.1016/j.ymeth.2007.01.009

Becker, G. (1978). *The mad genius controversy: A study in the sociology of deviance.* Beverly Hills, CA: Sage.

Becker, G. (2000). The association of creativity and psychopathology: Its cultural-historical origins. *Creativity Research Journal, 13*(1), 45–53.

Becker, G. (2014). A Socio-historical Overview of the Creativity–Pathology Connection from Antiquity to Contemporary Times. In J.C. Kaufman (Ed.), *Creativity and mental illness* (in press).

Beer, M.D. (1996). Psychosis: a history of the concept. *Compr Psychiatry, 37*(4), 273–91.

Benfey, O.T. (1958). August Kekule and the birth of the structural theory of organic chemistry in 1858. *Journal of Chemical Education, 35*, 21.

Bengtsson, S.L., Csikszentmihalyi, M. and Ullen, F. (2007). Cortical regions involved in the generation of musical structures during improvisation in pianists. *J Cogn Neurosci, 19*(5), 830–42. doi: 10.1162/jocn.2007.19.5.830

Beveridge, A. and Yorston, G. (1999). I drink, therefore I am: alcohol and creativity. *J R Soc Med, 92*(12), 646–8.

Bhattacharya, J. and Petsche, H. (2002). Shadows of artistry: cortical synchrony during perception and imagery of visual art. *Cognitive Brain Research, 13*(2), 179–86. doi: Pii S0926–6410(01)00110–0

Bogen, J.E. and Bogen, G.M. (1969). The other side of the brain III: The corpus callosum and creativity. *Bulletin of the Los Angeles Neurological Society, 34*, 191–220.

Boone, B.K. (1998). Neurophysiological assessment of executive functions. In B.L. Miller and J.L. Cummings (Eds), *The human frontal lobes: Functions and disorders* (pp. 247–60). New York: Guilford Press.

Borelius, M., Lindhardt, A. and Schalling, M. (2014). Help break the stigma against mental illness! *Nord J Psychiatry, 68*(4), 225–6. doi: 10.3109/08039488.2014.910365

Boring, E.G. (1950). *A history of experimental psychology* (2nd ed.). New York: Appleton-Century-Crofts.

Bouchard, T.J., Jr. and McGue, M. (1981). Familial studies of intelligence: a review. *Science, 212*(4498), 1055–9.

Bousman, C.A., Yung, A.R., Pantelis, C., Ellis, J.A., Chavez, R.A., Nelson, B., . . . Foley, D.L. (2013). Effects of NRG1 and DAOA genetic variation on transition to psychosis in individuals at ultra-high risk for psychosis. *Transl Psychiatry, 3*, e251. doi: 10.1038/tp.2013.23

Brand, S., Beck, J., Kalak, N., Gerber, M., Kirov, R., Puhse, U., . . . Holsboer-Trachsler, E. (2011). Dream Recall and Its Relationship to Sleep, Perceived Stress & Creativity Among Adolescents. *Journal of Adolescent Health, 49*(5), 525–31. doi: 10.1016/j.jadohealth.2011.04.004

Brunke, M. and Gilbert, M. (1992). Alcohol and creative writing. *Psychol Rep, 71*(2), 651–8.

Burch, G.S., Pavelis, C., Hemsley, D.R. and Corr, P.J. (2006). Schizotypy and creativity in visual artists. *Br J Psychol, 97*(Pt 2), 177–90. doi: 10.1348/000 712605X60030

Burke, B., Chrisler, J. and Devlin, A. (1989). The creative thinking, environmental frustration & self-concept of left- and right-handers. *Creativity Research Journal, 2*, 279–85.

Campbell, B.C. and Wang, S.S.H. (2012). Familial Linkage between Neuro-psychiatric Disorders and Intellectual Interests. *PLoS One, 7*(1). doi: ARTN e3040510.1371/journal.pone.0030405

Campbell, B.G. (1972). *Sexual selection and the descent of man, 1871–1971.* Chicago: Aldine Pub. Co.

Campbell, D.T. (1960). Blind Variation and Selective Retention in Creative Thought as in Other Knowledge Processes. *Psychological Review, 67*(6), 380–400. doi: 10.1037/H0040373

Campbell, D.T. (1974). Evolutionary epistemology. In P.A. Schilpp (Ed.), *The philosophy of Karl Popper* (pp. 413–63). La Salle, Ill.: Open Court.

Canesi, M., Rusconi, M.L., Isaias, I.U. and Pezzoli, G. (2012). Artistic productivity and creative thinking in Parkinson's disease. *Eur J Neurol, 19*(3), 468–72. doi: 10.1111/j.1468–1331.2011.03546.x

Canter, S. (1973). Personality traits in twins. In G. Claridge, S. Canter and W.I. Hume (Eds), *Personality differences and biological variations: A study of twins.* Oxford: Pergamon.

Carlsson, I., Wendt, P.E. and Risberg, J. (2000). On the neurobiology of creativity. Differences in frontal activity between high and low creative subjects. *Neuropsychologia, 38*(6), 873–85. doi: S0028-3932(99)00128-1 [pii]

Carra, G. and Barale, F. (2004). Cesare Lombroso, M.D., 1835–1909. *Am J Psychiatry, 161*(4), 624.

Carson, S.H., Peterson, J.B. and Higgins, D.M. (2005). Reliability, validity & factor structure of the creative achievement questionnaire. *Creativity Research Journal, 17*(1), 37–50.

Carter, H.D. (1932). Twin similarities in occupational interests. *Journal of educational psychology, 23*(9), 641.

Cattell, J.M. (1903). A statistical study of eminent men. *Popular Science Monthly, 62*, 359–77.

Cattell, R.B., Eber, H.W. and Tatsuoka, M.M. *Handbook for the sixteen personality factor questionnaire (16 PF) in clinical, educational, industrial and research psychology, for use with all forms of the test, by Raymond B. Cattell, Herbert W. Eber and Maurice M. Tatsuoka*: Champaign.

Chabris, C.F., Hebert, B.M., Benjamin, D.J., Beauchamp, J., Cesarini, D., van der Loos, M., ... Laibson, D. (2012). Most Reported Genetic Associations With General Intelligence Are Probably False Positives. *Psychological Science, 23*(11), 1314–23. doi: Doi 10.1177/0956797611435528

Champkin, J. (2011). Francis Galton centenary. *Significance, 8*(3), 121–121. doi: 10.1111/j.1740-9713.2011.00507.x

Chapman, J.P. and Chapman, L.J. (1987). Handedness of hypothetically psychosis-prone subjects. *J Abnorm Psychol, 96*(2), 89–93.

Chavez-Eakle, R.A., Lara, M.D.C. and Cruz-Fuentes, C. (2006). Personality: A possible bridge between creativity and psychopathology? *Creativity Research Journal, 18*(1), 27–38. doi: 10.1207/s15326934crj1801_4

Chavez-Eakle, R.A., Graff-Guerrero, A., Garcia-Reyna, J.C., Vaugier, V. and Cruz-Fuentes, C. (2007). Cerebral blood flow associated with creative performance: A comparative study. *Neuroimage, 38*(3), 519–28. doi: S1053-8119(07)00609-X [pii] 10.1016/j.neuroimage.2007.07.059

Cieslik, E.C., Zilles, K., Caspers, S., Roski, C., Kellermann, T.S., Jakobs, O., ... Eickhoff, S.B. (2013). Is there 'one' DLPFC in cognitive action control? Evidence for heterogeneity from co-activation-based parcellation. *Cerebral Cortex, 23*(11), 2677–89. doi: 10.1093/cercor/bhs256

Claridge, G. (2009). Preamble. *Personality and Individual Differences, 46*(8), 753–4. doi: 10.1016/j.paid.2009.01.022

Claridge, G. (2012). Study links creativity and mental illness. Retrieved 30 April, 2014, from http://www.bps.org.uk/news/research-links-creativity-and-mental-illness

Claridge, G. and McDonald, A. (2009). An investigation into the relationships between convergent and divergent thinking, schizotypy and autistic traits. *Personality and Individual Differences, 46*(8), 794–9. doi: 10.1016/j.paid.2009.01.018

Claridge, G., McCreery, C., Mason, O., Bentall, R., Boyle, G. and Slade, P. (1996). The factor structure of 'schizotypal' traits: A large replication study. *British Journal of Clinical Psychology, 35*, 103–15.

Cline, V.B., Richards, J.M. and Abe, C. (1962). The Validity of a Battery of Creativity Tests in a High-School Sample. *Educational and Psychological Measurement, 22*(4), 781–4. doi: 10.1177/001316446202200416

Colangeloa, N., Kerrb, B., Hallowellc, K., Huesmand, R. and Gaethe, J. (1992). The Iowa inventiveness inventory: Toward a measure of mechanical inventiveness. *Creativity Research Journal, 5*(2), 157–63.

Cole, T.J. (2000). Secular trends in growth. *The Proceedings of the Nutrition Society, 59*(2), 317–24.

Cox, C.M., Gillan, L.O., Livesay, R.H. and Terman, L.M. (1926). *The Early Mental Traits of Three Hundred Geniuses. [By] C.M. Cox, assised by Lela O. Gillan, Ruth Haines Livesay, Lewis M. Terman. [With tables.]*: pp. xxiii. 842. Stanford University Press: Stanford University: G.G. Harrap and Co.: London.

Crofts, H.S., Dalley, J.W., Collins, P., Van Denderen, J.C., Everitt, B.J., Robbins, T.W. and Roberts, A.C. (2001). Differential effects of 6-OHDA lesions of the frontal cortex and caudate nucleus on the ability to acquire an attentional set. *Cerebral Cortex, 11*(11), 1015–26.

Csikszentmihalyi, M. (1996). *Creativity: Flow and the psychology of discovery and invention.* New York: HarperCollins.

Cziko, G. (1995). *Without miracles: Universal selection theory and the second Darwinian revolution.* Cambridge, Mass.; London: MIT Press.

Damasio, A.R. (1994). *Descartes' error: Emotion, reason and the human brain.* New York: G.P. Putnam.

Darwin, C. (1859). *On the origin of species by means of natural selection.* London,: J. Murray.

Darwin, C. (1871). *The descent of man & selection in relation to sex. By Charles Darwin ... In two volumes...With illustrations*: London: John Murray.

De Manzano, O., Cervenka, S., Karabanov, A., Farde, L. and Ullen, F. (2010). Thinking outside a less intact box: Thalamic dopamine D2 receptor densities are negatively related to psychometric creativity in healthy individuals. *PLoS One, 5*(5), e10670. doi: 10.1371/journal.pone.0010670

De Souza, L.C., Volle, E., Bertoux, M., Czernecki, V., Funkiewiez, A., Allali, G., ... Levy, R. (2010). Poor creativity in frontotemporal dementia: A window into the neural bases of the creative mind. *Neuropsychologia, 48*(13), 3733–42. doi: 10.1016/j.neuropsychologia.2010.09.010

Del Giudice, M., Angeleri, R., Brizio, A. and Elena, M.R. (2010). The evolution of autistic-like and schizotypal traits: A sexual selection hypothesis. *Frontiers in Psychology, 1.* doi: 10.3389/fpsyg.2010.00041

Dennett, D.C. (1995). *Darwin's dangerous idea: Evolution and the meanings of life.* New York: Simon and Schuster.

Dias, M. (2010). A decade for psychiatric disorders. *Nature, 463*(7277), 9. doi: 463009a [pii]10.1038/463009a

Dietrich, A. (2004). The cognitive neuroscience of creativity. *Psychon Bull Rev, 11*(6), 1011–26.

Dietrich, A. (2007). Who's afraid of a cognitive neuroscience of creativity? *Methods, 42*(1), 22–27. doi: S1046–2023(06)00310–0 [pii]10.1016/j.ymeth.2006.12.009

Dietrich, A. and Kanso, R. (2010). A Review of EEG, ERP & Neuroimaging Studies of Creativity and Insight. *Psychological Bulletin, 136*(5), 822–48. doi: 10.1037/A0019749

Dollinger, S.J., Urban, K.K. and James, T.A. (2004). Creativity and openness: Further validation of two creative product measures. *Creativity Research Journal, 16*(1), 35–47.

Doughty, O.J., Lawrence, V.A., Al-Mousawi, A., Ashaye, K. and Done, D.J. (2009). Overinclusive thought and loosening of associations are not unique to schizophrenia and are produced in Alzheimer's dementia. *Cogn Neuropsychiatry,* 14(3), 149–64. doi: 10.1080/13546800902857918

Drago, V., Crucian, G.P., Foster, P.S., Cheong, J., Finney, G.R., Pisani, F. and Heilman, K.M. (2006). Lewy body dementia and creativity: Case report. *Neuropsychologia,* 44(14), 3011–15. doi: 10.1016/j.neuropsychologia.2006.05.030

Dragovic, M. and Hammond, G. (2005). Handedness in schizophrenia: a quantitative review of evidence. *Acta Psychiatr Scand, 111*(6), 410–19. doi: 10.1111/j. 1600–0447.2005.00519.x

Dudbridge, F. (2013). Power and Predictive Accuracy of Polygenic Risk Scores. *PLoS genetics, 9*(3), e1003348. doi: 10.1371/journal.pgen.1003348

Dunbar, K. (1995). How scientists really reason: Scientific reasoning in real-world laboratories. In R.J. Sternberg and J.E. Davidson (Eds), *The nature of insight* (pp. 365–95). Cambridge, Mass.: MIT Press.

Dykes, M. and Mcghie, A. (1976). Comparative-Study of Attentional Strategies of Schizophrenic and Highly Creative Normal Subjects. *British Journal of Psychiatry, 128*(Jan), 50–6.

Edelman, G.M. (1987). *Neural Darwinism: The theory of neuronal group selection.* New York: Basic Books.

Egerton, A., Mehta, M.A., Montgomery, A.J., Lappin, J.M., Howes, O.D., Reeves, S.J., ... Grasby, P.M. (2009). The dopaminergic basis of human behaviors: A review of molecular imaging studies. *Neurosci Biobehav Rev, 33*(7), 1109–32. doi: S0149–7634(09)00077–3 [pii] 10.1016/j.neubiorev.2009.05.005

Eisen, M.L. (1989). Assessing differences in children with learning disabilities and normally achieving students with a new measure of creativity. *J Learn Disabil, 22*(7), 462–4, 451.

Ellis, H. (1904). *A study of British Genius.* London: Hurst & Blackett.

Elsworth, J.D., Leahy, D.J., Roth, R.H. and Redmond, D.E., Jr (1987). Homovanillic acid concentrations in brain, CSF and plasma as indicators of central dopamine function in primates. *J Neural Transm, 68*(1–2), 51–62.

Ericsson, K.A., Krampe, R.T. and Teschromer, C. (1993). The Role of Deliberate Practice in the Acquisition of Expert Performance. *Psychological Review, 100*(3), 363–406. doi: 10.1037/0033–295x.100.3.363

Ericsson, K.A., Roring, R.W. and Nandagopal, K. (2007). Giftedness and evidence for reproducibly superior performance: an account based on the expert performance framework. *High Ability Studies, 18*(1), 3–56. doi: 10.1080/13598130701350593

Evans, L., Akiskal, H.S., Keck, P.E., Jr, McElroy, S.L., Sadovnick, A.D., Remick, R.A. and Kelsoe, J.R. (2005). Familiality of temperament in bipolar disorder: Support for a genetic spectrum. *J Affect Disord, 85*(1–2), 153–68. doi: 10.1016/j.jad.2003.10.015

Ewen, R.B. (1997). *Personality: A topical approach: theories, research, major controversies and emerging findings.* Mahwah, N.J.: L. Erlbaum Associates.

Eysenck, H.J. (1975). *Manual of the Eysenck Personality Questionnaire (Junior and Adult).* [S.l.]: Hodder & Stoughton.

Eysenck, H.J. (1981). *A Model for personality.* Berlin; New York: Springer-Verlag.

Eysenck, H.J. (1995). *Genius: The natural history of creativity.* Cambridge; New York: Cambridge University Press.

Eysenck, H.J. and Eysenck, S.B.G. (1976). *Psychoticism as a dimension for personality.* New York: Crane, Russak & Co.

Feist, G.J. (1998). A meta-analysis of personality in scientific and artistic creativity. *Pers Soc Psychol Rev, 2*(4), 290–309. doi: 10.1207/s15327957pspr0204_5

Fink, A. and Benedek, M. (2012). EEG alpha power and creative ideation. *Neurosci Biobehav Rev.* doi: 10.1016/j.neubiorev.2012.12.002

Fink, A., Graif, B. and Neubauer, A.C. (2009). Brain correlates underlying creative thinking: EEG alpha activity in professional vs. novice dancers. *Neuroimage, 46*(3), 854–62. doi: 10.1016/j.neuroimage.2009.02.036

Fink, A., Grabner, R.H., Benedek, M., Reishofer, G., Hauswirth, V., Fally, M., ... Neubauer, A.C. (2009). The creative brain: Investigation of brain activity during creative problem solving by means of EEG and FMRI. *Hum Brain Mapp, 30*(3), 734–48. doi: 10.1002/hbm.20538

Fink, A., Slamar-Halbedl, M., Unterrainer, H.F. and Weiss, E.M. (2012). Creativity: Genius, Madness, or a Combination of Both? *Psychology of Aesthetics Creativity and the Arts, 6*(1), 11–18. doi: 10.1037/A0024874

Finke, R.A. (1996). Imagery, creativity & emergent structure. *Conscious Cogn, 5*(3), 381–93. doi: 10.1006/ccog.1996.0024

Fitzgerald, M. (2004). *Autism and creativity: Is there a link between autism in men and exceptional ability?* Hove; New York: Brunner-Routledge.

Flaherty, A.W. (2005). Frontotemporal and dopaminergic control of idea generation and creative drive. *J Comp Neurol, 493*(1), 147–53. doi: 10.1002/cne.20768

Florida, R.L. (2002). *The rise of the creative class: And how it's transforming work, leisure, community and everyday life.* New York: Basic Books.

Fodor, E.M. and Carver, R.A. (2000). Achievement and power motives, performance feedback & creativity. *Journal of Research in Personality, 34*(4), 380–96. doi: 10.1006/jrpe.2000.2289

Folley, B.S. and Park, S. (2005). Verbal creativity and schizotypal personality in relation to prefrontal hemispheric laterality: A behavioral and near-infrared optical imaging study. *Schizophr Res, 80*(2–3), 271–82. doi: 10.1016/j.schres.2005.06.016

Forgeard, M. (2008). Linguistic styles of eminent writers suffering from unipolar and bipolar mood disorder. *Creativity Research Journal, 20*(1), 81–92. doi: 10.1080/10400410701842094

Forrest, D.W. (1974). *Francis Galton: The life and work of a Victorian genius.* London: Elek.

Frank, M.J. and Fossella, J.A. (2011). Neurogenetics and pharmacology of learning, motivation & cognition. *Neuropsychopharmacology, 36*(1), 133–52. doi: 10.1038/npp.2010.96

Funk, J.B., Chessare, J.B., Weaver, M.T. and Exley, A.R. (1993). Attention deficit hyperactivity disorder, creativity & the effects of methylphenidate. *Pediatrics, 91*(4), 816–19.

Futuyma, D.J. (2009). *Evolution* (2nd ed.). Sunderland, Mass.: Sinauer Associates.

Gabora, L. (2005). Creative thought as a nonDarwinian evolutionary process. *Journal of Creative Behavior, 39*(4), 262–83.

Galenson, D.W. (2006). *Old masters and young geniuses: The two life cycles of artistic creativity.* Princeton, N.J.; Oxford: Princeton University Press.

Galton, F. (1865). Hereditary Talent and Character. *Macmillan's Magazine, 12,* 157–66, 318–27.

Galton, F. (1869). *Hereditary Genius: An enquiry into its laws and consequences*: London.

Galton, F. (1874). *English men of science: Their nature and nurture*. London: Macmillan & Co.

Gamman, L. and Raein, M. (2010). Reviewing the art of crime – what, if anything, do criminals and artists/designers have in common? In D. Cropley (Ed.), *The dark side of creativity* (pp. 155–77). Cambridge: Cambridge University Press.

Gardner, H. (1993). *Creating minds: An anatomy of creativity seen through the lives of Freud, Einstein, Picasso, Stravinsky, Eliot, Graham & Gandhi*. New York: Basic Books.

Gazzaniga, M.S., Ivry, R.B. and Mangun, G.R. (2009). *Cognitive neuroscience: The biology of the mind* (3rd ed.). New York: W.W. Norton.

George, J.M. and Zhou, J. (2001). When openness to experience and conscientiousness are related to creative behavior: An interactional approach. *Journal of Applied Psychology, 86*(3), 513–24. doi: 10.1037//0021-9010.86.3.513

Gerard, A. (1774). *An essay on genius*. London: Printed for W. Strahan; T. Cadell; etc.

Getzels, J.W. and Jackson, P.W. (1962). *Creativity and intelligence: Explorations with gifted students*. New York: Wiley.

Ghadirian, A.M., Gregoire, P. and Kosmidis, H. (2000). Creativity and the evolution of psychopathologies. *Creativity Research Journal, 13*(2), 145–8.

Ghaemi, S.N. (2009). *A clinician's guide to statistics and epidemiology in mental health: Measuring truth and uncertainty*. Cambridge, UK; New York: Cambridge University Press.

Glover, J.A. and Tramel, S. (1976). Comparative levels of creative ability among students with and without behavior problems. *Psychol Rep, 38*(3 Pt 2), 1171–4.

Goel, V. and Vartanian, O. (2005). Dissociating the roles of right ventral lateral and dorsal lateral prefrontal cortex in generation and maintenance of hypotheses in set-shift problems. *Cerebral Cortex, 15*(8), 1170–7. doi: 10.1093/cercor/bhh217

Goertzel, V. (1965). *Cradles of Eminence*. [S.l.]: Constable.

Goldberg, T.E., Egan, M.F., Gscheidle, T., Coppola, R., Weickert, T., Kolachana, B.S., ... Weinberger, D.R. (2003). Executive subprocesses in working memory: Relationship to catechol-O-methyltransferase Val158Met genotype and schizophrenia. *Arch Gen Psychiatry, 60*(9), 889–96. doi: 10.1001/archpsyc.60.9.889

Gonen-Yaacovi, G., De Souza, L.C., Levy, R., Urbanski, M., Josse, G. and Volle, E. (2013). Rostral and caudal prefrontal contribution to creativity: A meta-analysis of functional imaging data. *Frontiers in Human Neuroscience, 7*. doi: 10.3389/fnhum.2013.00465

Goodwin, F.K. and Jamison, K.R. (2007). *Manic-Depressive Illness*. Oxford: Oxford University Press.

Gough, H.G. (1979). A creative personality scale for the Adjective Check List. *Journal of Personality and Social Psychology, 37*, 1398–405.

Gowan, J.C. (1963). Cradles of Eminence. *Gifted Child Quarterly, 7*(4), 185–185.

Graham, S. and Sheinker, A. (1980). Creative capabilities of learning-disabled and normal students. *Percept Mot Skills, 50*(2), 481–2.

Graña, C. (1964). *Bohemian versus bourgeois; French society and the French man of letters in the nineteenth century*. New York: Basic Books.

Gray, J.A. (1981). A critique of Eysenck's theory of personality. In H.J. Eysenck (Ed.), *A Model for personality*. Berlin; New York: Springer-Verlag.

Grigorenko, E., LaBuda, M.C. and Carter, A. (1992). Similarity in general cognitive ability, creativity and cognitive style in a sample of adolescent Russian twins. *Acta Geneticae Medicae et Gemellologiae: Twin Research, 41*(1), 65–72.

Grimes, D.A. and Schulz, K.F. (2012). False alarms and pseudo-epidemics: the limitations of observational epidemiology. *Obstet Gynecol, 120*(4), 920–27. doi: 10.1097/AOG.0b013e31826af61a

Guilford, J.P. (1950). Creativity. *American Psychologist, 5*(9), 444–54. doi: 10.1037/h0063487

Guilford, J.P. (1967). *The nature of human intelligence* (1967). New York: McGraw-Hill.

Haggard, P. (2008). Human volition: Towards a neuroscience of will. *Nat Rev Neurosci, 9*(12), 934–46. doi: 10.1038/nrn2497

Harrington, D.M. (1975). Effects of explicit instructions to 'be creative' on psychological meaning of divergent thinking test scores. *Journal of Personality, 43*, 434–54.

Healey, D. and Rucklidge, J.J. (2005). An exploration into the creative abilities of children with ADHD. *J Atten Disord, 8*(3), 88–95. doi: 10.1177/1087054705277198

Healey, D. and Rucklidge, J.J. (2006). An investigation into the relationship among ADHD symptomatology, creativity & neuropsychological functioning in children. *Child Neuropsychol, 12*(6), 421–38. doi: 10.1080/09297040600806086

Helson, R. (1999). Institute of personality assessment and research. In M.A. Runco and S. Pritzker (Eds), *Encyclopedia of Creativity* (pp. 71–9). San Diego: Academic Press.

Hennessy, B.A. (2010). The creativity-motivation connection. In J.C. Kaufman and R.J. Sternberg (Eds), *The Cambridge handbook of creativity* (pp. 342–65). Cambridge; New York: Cambridge University Press.

Herbert, P.S., Jr (1959). Creativity and mental illness: A study of 60 creative patients who needed hospitalization. *Psychiatr Q, 33*, 534–47.

Hickey, M. (2001). An application of Amabile's consensual assessment technique for rating the creativity of children's musical compositions. *Journal of Research in Music Education, 49*(3), 234–44. doi: Doi 10.2307/3345709

Hill, A.B. (1965). The Environment and Disease: Association or Causation? *Proc R Soc Med, 58*, 295–300.

Hirschowitz, J., Kolevzon, A. and Garakani, A. (2010). The pharmacological treatment of bipolar disorder: The question of modern advances. *Harv Rev Psychiatry, 18*(5), 266–78. doi: 10.3109/10673229.2010.507042

Hobson, J.A., Hobson, R.P., Malik, S., Bargiota, K. and Calo, S. (2013). The relation between social engagement and pretend play in autism. *Br J Dev Psychol, 31*(Pt 1), 114–27. doi: 10.1111/j.2044-835X.2012.02083.x

Holden, R.B. (2010). Face validity. In I.B. Weiner and W.E. Craighead (Eds), *The Corsini encyclopedia of psychology* (4th ed., pp. 637–38). Hoboken, N.J.: Wiley.

Hoppe, K.D. and Kyle, N.L. (1990). Dual brain, creativity & health. *Creativity Research Journal, 3*(2), 150–7. doi: 10.1080/10400419009534348

Howard-Jones, P.A., Blakemore, S.J., Samuel, E.A., Summers, I.R. and Claxton, G. (2005). Semantic divergence and creative story generation: An fMRI investigation. *Brain Res Cogn Brain Res, 25*(1), 240–50. doi: S0926–6410(05)00163–1 [pii] 10.1016/j.cogbrainres.2005.05.013

Howard-Jones, P.A. and Murray, S. (2003). Ideational productivity, focus of attention & context. *Creativity Research Journal, 15*(2–3), 153–66.

Howick, J., Chalmers, I., Glasziou, P., Greenhalgh, T., Heneghan, C., Liberati, A., Moschetti, I., Phillips, B. and Thornton, T. (2011). Explanation of the 2011 Oxford Centre for Evidence-Based Medicine (OCEBM) Levels of Evidence (Background Document). Oxford Centre for Evidence-Based Medicine. http://www.cebm.net/

index.aspx?o=5653Retrieved9August2014,fromhttp://www.cebm.net/wp-content/uploads/2014/06/CEBM-Levels-of-Evidence-Background-Document-2.1.pdf

Humphreys, K., Grankvist, A., Leu, M., Hall, P., Liu, J., Ripatti, S., ... Magnusson, P.K.E. (2011). The Genetic Structure of the Swedish Population. *PLoS One, 6*(8), e22547. doi: 10.1371/journal.pone.0022547

Hunter, S.T., Bedell, K.E. and Mumford, M.D. (2007). Climate for creativity: A quantitative review. *Creativity Research Journal, 19*(1), 69–90.

Jamison, K.R. (1989). Mood Disorders and Patterns of Creativity in British Writers and Artists. *Psychiatry-Interpersonal and Biological Processes, 52*(2), 125–34.

Jamison, K.R. (1996). *Touched with Fire: Manic-depressive Illness and the Artistic Temperament*: Simon & Schuster Ltd.

Jamison, K.R. (2000). Reply to Louis A. Sass: 'Schizophrenia, Modernism and the "creative imagination"'. *Creativity Research Journal, 13*(1), 75–6.

Jaracz, J., Patrzala, A. and Rybakowski, J.K. (2012). Creative Thinking Deficits in Patients With Schizophrenia Neurocognitive Correlates. *Journal of Nervous and Mental Disease, 200*(7), 588–93. doi: 10.1097/NMD.0b013e31825bfc49

Jarosz, A.F., Colflesh, G.J. and Wiley, J. (2012). Uncorking the muse: Alcohol intoxication facilitates creative problem solving. *Conscious Cogn, 21*(1), 487–93. doi: 10.1016/j.concog.2012.01.002

Jauk, E., Benedek, M. and Neubauer, A.C. (2012). Tackling creativity at its roots: Evidence for different patterns of EEG alpha activity related to convergent and divergent modes of task processing. *International Journal of Psychophysiology, 84*(2), 219–25. doi: 10.1016/j.ijpsycho.2012.02.012

Johnson, S.L., Edge, M.D., Holmes, M.K. and Carver, C.S. (2012). The behavioral activation system and mania. *Annu Rev Clin Psychol, 8*, 243–67. doi: 10.1146/annurev-clinpsy-032511-143148

Jolley, R.P., O'Kelly, R., Barlow, C.M. and Jarrold, C. (2013). Expressive drawing ability in children with autism. *Br J Dev Psychol, 31*(Pt 1), 143–9. doi: 10.1111/bjdp.12008

Juda, A. (1949). The relationship between highest mental capacity and psychic abnormalities. *Am J Psychiatry, 106*(4), 296–307.

Jung-Beeman, M., Bowden, E.M., Haberman, J., Frymiare, J.L., Arambel-Liu, S., Greenblatt, R., ... Kounios, J. (2004). Neural activity when people solve verbal problems with insight. *PLoS Biol, 2*(4), E97. doi: 10.1371/journal.pbio.0020097

Jung, R.E., Gasparovic, C., Chavez, R.S., Flores, R.A., Smith, S.M., Caprihan, A. and Yeo, R.A. (2009). Biochemical support for the 'threshold' theory of creativity: A magnetic resonance spectroscopy study. *J Neurosci, 29*(16), 5319–25. doi: 29/16/5319 [pii] 10.1523/JNEUROSCI.0588–09.2009

Jung, R.E., Segall, J.M., Jeremy Bockholt, H., Flores, R.A., Smith, S.M., Chavez, R.S. and Haier, R.J. (2009). Neuroanatomy of creativity. *Hum Brain Mapp, 31*(3), 398–409. doi: 10.1002/hbm.20874

Jung, R.E., Grazioplene, R., Caprihan, A., Chavez, R.S. and Haier, R.J. (2010). White matter integrity, creativity & psychopathology: disentangling constructs with diffusion tensor imaging. *PLoS One, 5*(3), e9818. doi: 10.1371/journal.pone.0009818

Jung, W.H., Jang, J.H., Byun, M.S., An, S.K. and Kwon, J.S. (2010). Structural brain alterations in individuals at ultra-high risk for psychosis: a review of magnetic resonance imaging studies and future directions. *J Korean Med Sci, 25*(12), 1700–9. doi: 10.3346/jkms.2010.25.12.1700

Karlsson, J.L. (1970). Genetic association of giftedness and creativity with schizophrenia. *Hereditas, 66,* 177–82.

Karlsson, J.L. (1984). Creative Intelligence in Relatives of Mental-Patients. *Hereditas, 100*(1), 83–6.

Karlsson, J.L. (1999). Relation of mathematical ability to psychosis in Iceland. *Clin Genet, 56*(6), 447–449.

Katz, A.N. (1997). Creativity in the cerebral hemispheres. In M.A. Runco (Ed.), *The creativity research handbook* (pp. 203–26). Cresskill, N.J.: Hampton Press.

Kauffman, C., Grunebaum, H., Cohler, B. and Gamer, E. (1979). Superkids: Competent children of psychotic mothers. *Am J Psychiatry, 136*(11), 1398–402.

Kaufman, J.C. (2001). The Sylvia Plath Effect: Mental Illness in Eminent Creative Writers. *Journal of Creative Behavior,* 35(1), 37–50.

Kaufman, J.C. and Beghetto, R.A. (2009). Beyond Big and Little: The Four C Model of Creativity. *Review of General Psychology, 13*(1), 1–12. doi: 10.1037/A0013688

Kaufman, J.C. and Sternberg, R.J. (2010). *The Cambridge handbook of creativity.* Cambridge: Cambridge University Press.

Kaufman, J.C., Plucker, J.A. and Baer, J. (2008). *Essentials of creativity assessment.* Hoboken, N.J.: Wiley.

Kaufman, J.C., Baer, J., Cole, J.C. and Sexton, J.D. (2008). A comparison of expert and nonexpert raters using the consensual assessment technique. *Creativity Research Journal, 20*(2), 171–8. doi: 10.1080/10400410802059929

Kaufman, J.C., Cole, J.C. and Baer, J. (2009). The Construct of Creativity: Structural Model for Self-Reported Creativity Ratings. *Journal of Creative Behavior, 43*(2), 119–34.

Kayser, M. (2013). Editors' Pick: Mad and genius in the same gene? *Investig Genet,* 4(1), 14. doi: 10.1186/2041-2223-4-14

Keefe, J.A. and Magaro, P.A. (1980). Creativity and Schizophrenia – an Equivalence of Cognitive Processing. *Journal of Abnormal Psychology, 89*(3), 390–8.

Keri, S. (2009). Genes for psychosis and creativity: A promoter polymorphism of the neuregulin 1 gene is related to creativity in people with high intellectual achievement. *Psychol Sci, 20*(9), 1070–3. doi: PSCI2398 [pii] 10.1111/j.1467-9280.2009.02398.x

Kidner, D. (1976). Creativity and Socialization as Predictors of Abnormality. *Psychol Rep, 39*(3), 966–966.

Kim, D., Raine, A., Triphon, N. and Green, M.F. (1992). Mixed Handedness and Features of Schizotypal Personality in a Nonclinical Sample. *Journal of Nervous and Mental Disease, 180*(2), 133–5. doi: 10.1097/00005053-199202000-00012

Kim, K.H. (2005). Can Only Intelligent People Be Creative? *Journal of Secondary Gifted Education, XVI*(2–3), 57–66.

Kim, K.H., Cramond, B. and VanTassel-Baska, J. (2010). The relationship between creativity and intelligence. In J.C. Kaufman and R.J. Sternberg (Eds), *The Cambridge handbook of creativity* (pp. 395–412). Cambridge; New York: Cambridge University Press.

Kinney, D.K., Richards, R., Lowing, P.A., LeBlanc, D., Zimbalist, M.E. and Harlan, P. (2000). Creativity in offspring of schizophrenic and control parents: An adoption study. *Creativity Research Journal, 13*(1), 17–25.

Klimesch, W. (1999). EEG alpha and theta oscillations reflect cognitive and memory performance: A review and analysis. *Brain Res Brain Res Rev, 29*(2–3), 169–95.

Klimesch, W. (2012). Alpha-band oscillations, attention & controlled access to stored information. *Trends Cogn Sci, 16*(12), 606–17. doi: 10.1016/j.tics.2012. 10.007

Kline, P. and Cooper, C. (1986). Psychoticism and creativity. *J Genet Psychol, 147*(2), 183–8. doi: 10.1080/00221325.1986.9914492

Knepper, P. and Ystehede, P. (2013). *The Cesare Lombroso handbook.* London: Routledge.

Kowatari, Y., Lee, S.H., Yamamura, H., Nagamori, Y., Levy, P., Yamane, S. and Yamamoto, M. (2009). Neural networks involved in artistic creativity. *Hum Brain Mapp, 30*(5), 1678–90. doi: 10.1002/hbm.20633

Koza, J.R. (1992). *Genetic programming: On the programming of computers by means of natural selection.* Cambridge, Mass.; London: MIT.

Kozbelt, A. (2008). Longitudinal Hit Ratios of Classical Composers: Reconciling 'Darwinian' and Expertise Acquisition Perspectives on Lifespan Creativity. *Psychology of Aesthetics, Creativity and the Arts, 2*(4), 221–35.

Kozbelt, A., Beghetto, R.A. and Runco, M.A. (2010). Theories of creativity. In J.C. Kaufman and R.J. Sternberg (Eds), *The Cambridge handbook of creativity* (pp. 20–47). Cambridge; New York: Cambridge University Press.

Kraepelin, E. (1883). *Compendium der Psychiatrie zum Gebrauche für Studirende und Aerzte.* Leipzig: Abel.

Kuhn, T.S. (1962). *The structure of scientific revolutions.* Chicago; London: University of Chicago Press.

Kurian, M.A., Gissen, P., Smith, M., Heales, S., Jr and Clayton, P.T. (2011). The monoamine neurotransmitter disorders: An expanding range of neurological syndromes. *Lancet Neurol, 10*(8), 721–33. doi: 10.1016/S1474–4422(11)70141–7

Kyaga, S. (2014). *Creativity and psychopathology.* (PhD), Karolinska Institutet. Retrieved from http://hdl.handle.net/10616/41931

Kyaga, S. and Liberg, B. (2010). *Meta-analysis of functional neuroimaging studies investigating insight.* Manuscript

Kyaga, S., Lichtenstein, P., Boman, M., Hultman, C., Langstrom, N. and Landen, M. (2011). Creativity and mental disorder: family study of 300 000 people with severe mental disorder. *Br J Psychiatry, 199*, 373–9. doi: bjp.bp.110.085316 [pii] 10.1192/bjp.bp.110.085316

Kyaga, S., Landen, M., Boman, M., Hultman, C.M., Langstrom, N. and Lichtenstein, P. (2012). Mental illness, suicide and creativity: 40-Year prospective total population study. *J Psychiatr Res.* doi: S0022–3956(12)00280–4 [pii] 10.1016/j. jpsychires.2012.09.010

Kyaga, S., Landen, M., Boman, M., Hultman, C.M., Langstrom, N. and Lichtenstein, P. (2013). Mental illness, suicide and creativity: 40-year prospective total population study. *J Psychiatr Res, 47*(1), 83–90. doi: 10.1016/j.jpsychires.2012.09.010

Kyaga, S., Fogelberg, J., Sellgren, C. and Landén, M. (2014). *Cognitive and biological markers for creative achievement.* Poster presented at the The Molecular Basis of Brain Disorders, Miami, United States of America.

La Caze, A. (2009). Evidence-Based Medicine Must Be …. *Journal of Medicine and Philosophy, 34*(5), 509–27 doi: 10.1093/jmp/jhp034

Lang, A.R., Verret, L.D. and Watt, C. (1984). Drinking and creativity: objective and subjective effects. *Addict Behav, 9*(4), 395–9.

Lange-Eichbaum, W. (1928). *Genie - Irrsinn und Ruhm.* München: Ernst Reinhardt Verlag.

Lange-Eichbaum, W. and Paul, M.E. (1931). *[Das Genie-Problem.] The Problem of Genius ... Translated by Eden and Cedar Paul*: pp. xix, 187. Kegan Paul & Co.: London.

Lapp, W.M., Collins, R.L. and Izzo, C.V. (1994). On the enhancement of creativity by alcohol: Pharmacology or expectation? *Am J Psychol, 107*(2), 173–206.

Lauronen, E., Veijola, J., Isohanni, I., Jones, P.B., Nieminen, P. and Isohanni, M. (2004). Links between creativity and mental disorder. *Psychiatry-Interpersonal and Biological Processes, 67*(1), 81–98. doi: 10.1521/psyc.67.1.81.31245

Lee, H.C., Tsai, S.Y. and Lin, H.C. (2007). Seasonal variations in bipolar disorder admissions and the association with climate: A population-based study. *J Affect Disord, 97*(1–3), 61–9. doi: 10.1016/j.jad.2006.06.026

Lehman, H. (1947). National Differences in Creativity. *American Journal of Sociology, 52*, 475–88.

Lélut, L.F. (1836). *Du démon de Socrate*. Paris: Trinquart.

Lenzenweger, M.F. (2010). *Schizotypy and schizophrenia: The view from experimental psychopathology*. New York; London: Guilford.

Leonard, T.C. (2009). Origins of the myth of social Darwinism: The ambiguous legacy of Richard Hofstadter's Social Darwinism in American Thought. *Journal of Economic Behavior and Organization, 71*(1), 37–51. doi: 10.1016/j.jebo.2007.11.004

Lim, W. and Plucker, J.A. (2001). Creativity through a lens of social responsibility: Implicit theories of creativity with Korean samples. *Journal of Creative Behavior, 35*(2), 115–30.

Limb, C.J. and Braun, A.R. (2008). Neural substrates of spontaneous musical performance: An FMRI study of jazz improvisation. *PLoS One, 3*(2), e1679. doi: 10.1371/journal.pone.0001679

Linney, Y.M., Murray, R.M., Peters, E.R., MacDonald, A.M., Rijsdijk, F. and Sham, P.C. (2003). A quantitative genetic analysis of schizotypal personality traits. *Psychological medicine, 33*(5), 803–16.

Loewenberg, R.D. (1950). Wilhelm Lange-Eichbaum and 'The Problem of Genius'. *Am J Psychiatry, 106*, 927–8.

Lombroso, C. (1891). *The man of genius*. [S.l.]: Scott.

Lombroso, C. (1911). *Criminal Man*. New York; London: G.P. Putnam's Sons.

Lowe, G. (1994). Group differences in alcohol-creativity interactions. *Psychol Rep, 75*(3 Pt 2), 1635–8.

Ludwig, A.M. (1990). Alcohol input and creative output. *Br J Addict, 85*(7), 953–63.

Ludwig, A.M. (1992). Creative Achievement and Psychopathology – Comparison among Professions. *American Journal of Psychotherapy, 46*(3), 330–56.

Ludwig, A.M. (1994). Mental-Illness and Creative Activity in Female Writers. *American Journal of Psychiatry, 151*(11), 1650–6.

Ludwig, A.M. (1995). *The price of greatness: Resolving the creativity and madness controversy*. New York; London: Guilford Press.

MacDougall, A.K. and Montgomerie, R. (2003). Assortative mating by carotenoid-based plumage colour: A quality indicator in American goldfinches, Carduelis tristis. *Naturwissenschaften, 90*(10), 464–7. doi: 10.1007/s00114–003–0459–7

Mackinnon, D.W. (1960). The Highly Effective Individual. *Teachers College Record, 61*(7), 367–78.

Mackinnon, D.W. (1965). Personality and the Realization of Creative Potential. *American Psychologist, 20*(4), 273–81. doi: 10.1037/H0022403

Maj, M. and Ferro, M. (Eds) (2002). *Anthology of Italian Psychiatric Texts*. World Psychiatric Association. New York: Wiley.

Martindale, C. and Hines, D. (1975). Creativity and Cortical Activation during Creative, Intellectual and Eeg Feedback Tasks. *Biological Psychology, 3*(2), 91–100.

Mashal, N., Faust, M., Hendler, T. and Jung-Beeman, M. (2007). An fMRI investigation of the neural correlates underlying the processing of novel metaphoric expressions. *Brain Lang, 100*(2), 115–26. doi: S0093-934X(05)00309-3 [pii] 10.1016/j.bandl.2005.10.005

Mason, O. and Claridge, G. (2006). The Oxford–Liverpool Inventory of Feelings and Experiences (O-LIFE): Further description and extended norms. *Schizophr Res, 82*(2–3), 203–11. doi: S0920-9964(05)01391-5 [pii] 10.1016/j.schres.2005.12.845

Mathisen, G.E. and Einarsen, S. (2004). A review of instruments assessing creative and innovative environments within organizations. *Creativity Research Journal, 16*(1), 119–40. doi: 10.1207/s15326934crj1601_12

Maudsley, H. (1908). *Heredity, variation and genius*. [S.l.]: Bale, Sons & Danielsson.

Mayer, W. (1953). In memoriam: Robert Gaupp, 1870–1953. *Am J Psychiatry, 110*(6), 480.

McCrae, R.R. (1987). Creativity, Divergent Thinking & Openness to Experience. *Journal of Personality and Social Psychology, 52*(6), 1258–65.

McCrae, R.R. and John, O.P. (1992). An introduction to the five-factor model and its applications. *J Pers, 60*(2), 175–215.

McCrae, R.R. and Costa Jr, P.T. (2010). *NEO Inventories: Professional manual*. Lutz, FL: Psychological Assessment Resources, Inc.

McIntosh, A.M., Munoz Maniega, S., Lymer, G.K., McKirdy, J., Hall, J., Sussmann, J.E., ... Lawrie, S.M. (2008). White matter tractography in bipolar disorder and schizophrenia. *Biol Psychiatry, 64*(12), 1088–92. doi: 10.1016/j.biopsych.2008.07.026

McNeil, T.F. (1971). Prebirth and postbirth influence on the relationship between creative ability and recorded mental illness. *J Pers, 39*(3), 391–406.

Mednick, S.A. (1962). The Associative Basis of the Creative Process. *Psychological Review, 69*(3), 220–32. doi: 10.1037/H0048850

Mednick, S.A. (1968). The remote associates test. *Journal of Creative Behaviour, 2*, 213–14.

Meehl, P.E. (1992). Cliometric Metatheory – the Actuarial Approach to Empirical, History-Based Philosophy of Science. *Psychol Rep, 71*(2), 339–467.

Merriman, C. (1924). The intellectual resemblance of twins. *Psychological Monographs, 33*(5), i–57.

Miller, B.L., Cummings, J., Mishkin, F., Boone, K., Prince, F., Ponton, M. and Cotman, C. (1998). Emergence of artistic talent in frontotemporal dementia. *Neurology, 51*(4), 978–82.

Miller, G.F. (2000). *The mating mind: How sexual choice shaped the evolution of human nature* (1st ed.). New York: Doubleday.

Miller, G.F. and Tal, I.R. (2007). Schizotypy versus openness and intelligence as predictors of creativity. *Schizophr Res, 93*(1–3), 317–24. doi: 10.1016/j.schres.2007.02.007

Moher, D., Liberati, A., Tetzlaff, J., Altman, D.G. and Group, P. (2009). Preferred reporting items for systematic reviews and meta-analyses: The PRISMA statement. *BMJ, 339*, b2535. doi: 10.1136/bmj.b2535

194   *References*

Moran, S. and John-Steiner, V. (2003). Creativity in the making: Vygotsky's contemporary contribution to the dialectic of development and creativity. In R.K. Keith Sawyer, V. John-Steiner, S. Moran, R.J. Sternberg, D.H. Feldman, J. Nakamura and M. Csikszentmihalyi (Eds), *Creativity and Development* (pp. 61–90). New York: Oxford University Press.

Motto, A.L. and Clark, J.R. (1992). The Paradox of Genius and Madness: Seneca and his influence. *Cuadernos de Filología Clásica. Estudios latinos, 2,* 189–200.

Mraz, W. and Runco, M.A. (1994). Suicide ideation and creative problem solving. *Suicide Life Threat Behav, 24*(1), 38–47.

Muntaner, C., Tien, A.Y., Eaton, W.W. and Garrison, R. (1991). Occupational characteristics and the occurrence of psychotic disorders. *Soc Psychiatry Psychiatr Epidemiol, 26*(6), 273–80.

Murphy, C. (2009). The link between artistic creativity and psychopathology: Salvador Dali. *Personality and Individual Differences, 46*(8), 765–74. doi: 10.1016/j.paid.2009.01.020

Murphy, M., Runco, M.A., Acar, S. and Reiter-Palmon, R. (2013). Reanalysis of genetic data and rethinking dopamine's relationship with creativity. *Creativity Research Journal, 25*(1), 147–8. doi: http://dx.doi.org/10.1080/10400419.2013.752305

Murray, H.A. (1938). *Explorations in personality: A clinical and experimental study of fifty men of college age.* New York: Oxford University Press.

Nelson, B. (2007). Its Own Reward: A Phenomological Study of Artistic Creativity. *Journal of Phenomological Psychology, 38,* 217–55.

Nelson, B. and Rawlings, D. (2008). Relating Schizotypy and Personality to the Phenomenology of Creativity. *Schizophr Bull.* doi: sbn098 [pii] 10.1093/schbul/sbn098

Nelson, B., Fornito, A., Harrison, B.J., Yucel, M., Sass, L.A., Yung, A.R., ... McGorry, P.D. (2009). A disturbed sense of self in the psychosis prodrome: Linking phenomenology and neurobiology. *Neurosci Biobehav Rev, 33*(6), 807–17. doi: 10.1016/j.neubiorev.2009.01.002

Nettle, D. (2006). Schizotypy and mental health amongst poets, visual artists & mathematicians. *Journal of Research in Personality, 40,* 876–90.

Nettle, D. and Clegg, H. (2006). Schizotypy, creativity and mating success in humans. *Proc Biol Sci, 273*(1586), 611–15. doi: Y12623T706452278 [pii] 10.1098/rspb.2005.3349

Nicol, J.J. and Long, B. (1996). Creativity and percieved stress of female music therapists and hobbyists. *Creativity Research Journal, 9*(1), 1–10.

Nichols, R.C. (1978). Twin Studies of Ability, Personality and Interests. *Homo, 29*(3), 158–73.

Noble, E.P., Runco, M.A. and Ozkaragoz, T.Z. (1993). Creativity in alcoholic and nonalcoholic families. *Alcohol, 10*(4), 317–22.

Nordau, M.S. (1892/1993). *Degeneration.* Lincoln, Neb.; London: University of Nebraska Press.

Nowakowska, C., Strong, C.M., Santosa, C.M., Wang, P.W. and Ketter, T.A. (2005). Temperamental commonalities and differences in euthymic mood disorder patients, creative controls & healthy controls. *J Affect Disord, 85*(1–2), 207–15. doi: S0165032704000230 [pii] 10.1016/j.jad.2003.11.012

Owen, G.S., Cutting, J. and David, A.S. (2007). Are people with schizophrenia more logical than healthy volunteers? *Br J Psychiatry, 191,* 453–4. doi: 191/5/453 [pii] 10.1192/bjp.bp.107.037309

Paget, K.D. (1979). Creativity and its correlates in emotionally disturbed preschool children. *Psychol Rep, 44*(2), 595–8.

Papworth, M.A. and James, I.A. (2003). Creativity and mood: Towards a model of cognitive mediation. *Journal of Creative Behavior, 37*(1), 1–16.

Pearson, K. (1914). *The life, letters and labours of Francis Galton.* Cambridge: Cambridge University Press.

Pennebaker, J.W. (1997). Writing about emotional experiences as a therapeutic process. *Psychological Science, 8*, 162–6.

Peterson, J.M. and Lansky, L.M. (1974). Left-Handedness among Architects – Facts and Speculation. *Perceptual and Motor Skills, 38*(2), 547–50.

Peterson, J.M. and Lansky, L.M. (1977). Left-Handedness among Architects – Partial Replication and Some New Data. *Perceptual and Motor Skills, 45*(3), 1216–18.

Pezzullo, T.R. (1971). The genetic components of verbal divergent thinking and short term memory. *Dissertation Abstracts International, 32*(1-A), 252–3.

Phares, E.J. (1991). *Introduction to personality* (3rd ed.). New York: HarperCollins.

Phillips, R.H. (1982). Mood, creativity and psychotherapeutic participation of patients receiving lithium. *Psychosomatics, 23*(1), 81–7. doi: 10.1016/S0033-3182(82)70816-3

Pies, R. (2007). The historical roots of the 'bipolar spectrum': Did Aristotle anticipate Kraepelin's broad concept of manic-depression? *J Affect Disord, 100*(1–3), 7–11. doi: 10.1016/j.jad.2006.08.034

Plato. (2005). *Phaedrus* (C.J. Rowe, Trans.). London: Penguin.

Plomin, R. (2008). *Behavioral genetics* (5th ed.). New York: Worth Publishers.

Plomin, R., DeFries, J.C., Knopik, V.S. and Neiderhiser, J.M. (2012). *Behavioral genetics: A primer* (6th ed.). US: Worth Publishers.

Plucker, J.A. (1999). Is the proof in the pudding? Reanalyses of Torrance's (1958 to present) longitudinal data. *Creativity Research Journal, 12*(2), 103–14. doi: 10.1207/s15326934crj1202_3

Plucker, J.A. and Dana, R.Q. (1998). Creativity of undergraduates with and without family history of alcohol and other drug problems. *Addict Behav, 23*(5), 711–14. doi: 10.1016/S0306-4603(98)00024-0

Plucker, J.A. and Makel, M.C. (2010). Assessment of creativity. In J.C. Kaufman and R.J. Sternberg (Eds), *The Cambridge handbook of creativity* (pp. 48–73). Cambridge; New York: Cambridge University Press.

Plucker, J.A., Beghetto, R.A. and Dow, G.T. (2004). Why isn't creativity more important to educational psychologists? Potentials, pitfalls & future directions in creativity research. *Educational Psychologist, 39*(2), 83–96. doi: 10.1207/s15326985ep3902_1

Plucker, J.A., Runco, M.A. and Lim, W. (2006). Predicting ideational behavior from divergent thinking and discretionary time on task. *Creativity Research Journal, 18*(1), 55–63. doi: 10.1207/s15326934crj1801_7

Poincaré, H. and Halsted, G.B. (1913). *The foundations of science; Science and hypothesis, The value of science, Science and method.* New York and Garrison, N.Y.: Science Press.

Popper, K. (2002). *Conjectures and refutations: The growth of scientific knowledge.* London: Routledge.

Post, F. (1994). Creativity and psychopathology. A study of 291 world-famous men. *Br J Psychiatry, 165*(2), 22–34.

Post, F. (1996). Verbal creativity, depression and alcoholism. An investigation of one hundred American and British writers. *Br J Psychiatry, 168*(5), 545–55.

Prabhu, V., Sutton, C. and Sauser, W. (2008). Creativity and certain personality traits: Understanding the mediating effect of intrinsic motivation. *Creativity Research Journal, 20*(1), 53–66. doi: 10.1080/10400410701841955

Preti, A., De Biasi, F. and Miotto, P. (2001). Musical creativity and suicide. *Psychol Rep, 89*(3), 719–27.

Preti, A. and Miotto, P. (1999). Suicide among eminent artists. *Psychol Rep, 84*(1), 291–301. doi: 10.2466/Pr0.84.1.291-301

Preti, A., Sardu, C. and Piga, A. (2007). Mixed-handedness is associated with the reporting of psychotic-like beliefs in a non-clinical Italian sample. *Schizophr Res, 92*(1–3), 15–23. doi: 10.1016/j.schres.2007.01.028

Preti, A. and Vellante, M. (2007). Creativity and psychopathology: Higher rates of psychosis proneness and nonright-handedness among creative artists compared to same age and gender peers. *J Nerv Ment Dis, 195*(10), 837–45. doi: 10.1097/NMD.0b013e3181568180

Pring, L., Ryder, N., Crane, L. and Hermelin, B. (2012). Creativity in savant artists with autism. *Autism, 16*(1), 45–57. doi: 10.1177/1362361311403783

Quetelet, A. and Beamish, R. (1839). *Popular instructions on the calculation of probabilities.* London: J. Weale.

Ramey, C.H. and Weisberg, R.W. (2004). The 'poetical activity' of Emily Dickinson: A further test of the hypothesis that affective disorders foster creativity. *Creativity Research Journal, 16*(2–3), 173–85. doi: DOI 10.1207/s15326934crj1602and3_3

Razumnikova, O.M. (2007). Creativity related cortex activity in the remote associates task. *Brain Research Bulletin, 73*(1–3), 96–102. doi: 10.1016/j.brainresbull.2007.02.008

Reuter, M., Roth, S., Holve, K. and Hennig, J. (2006). Identification of first candidate genes for creativity: A pilot study. *Brain Res, 1069*(1), 190–7. doi: S0006–8993(05)01649–5 [pii] 10.1016/j.brainres.2005.11.046

Reznikoff, M., Domino, G., Bridges, C. and Honeyman, M. (1973). Creative abilities in identical and fraternal twins. *Behavior Genetics, 3*(4), 365–77.

Rhodes, M. (1987). An analysis of creativity. In S.G. Isaksen (Ed.), *Frontiers of creativity research: Beyond the basics* (pp. 216–22). Buffalo, N.Y.: Bearly Ltd.

Richards, R. (2007). Everyday creativity: Our hidden potential. In R. Richards (Ed.), *Everyday creativity and new views of human nature: Psychological, social and spiritual perspectives* (pp. 22–53). Washington, D.C.: American Psychological Association.

Richards, R., Kinney, D.K., Lunde, I., Benet, M. and Merzel, A.P. (1988). Creativity in manic-depressives, cyclothymes, their normal relatives & control subjects. *J Abnorm Psychol, 97*(3), 281–8.

Ritchie, T. and Noble, E.P. (2003). Association of seven polymorphisms of the D2 dopamine receptor gene with brain receptor-binding characteristics. *Neurochem Res, 28*(1), 73–82.

Rodrigue, A.L. and Perkins, D.R. (2012). Divergent Thinking Abilities Across the Schizophrenic Spectrum and Other Psychological Correlates. *Creativity Research Journal, 24*, 163–8.

Root-Bernstein, R.S., Bernstein, M.G. and Garnier, H. (1993). Identification of scientists making long-term, high-impact contributions, with notes on their methods of working. *Creativity Research Journal, 6*, 329–43.

Rosen, G. (1980). *Madness in society: Chapters in the historical sociology of mental illness* (Phoenix ed.). Chicago: University of Chicago.

Rothenberg, A. (1983). Psychopathology and creative cognition. A comparison of hospitalized patients, Nobel laureates & controls. *Arch Gen Psychiatry, 40*(9), 937–42.

Rothenberg, A. (1995). Creativity and affective illness: An objection. *Percept Mot Skills, 80*(1), 161–2.

Rothenberg, A. (2001). Bipolar illness, creativity & treatment. *Psychiatr Q, 72*(2), 131–47.

Rothman, K.J. (2012). *Epidemiology: An introduction* (2nd ed.). New York: Oxford University Press.

Rothman, K.J., Greenland, S. and Lash, T.L. (2008). *Modern epidemiology* (3rd ed.). Philadelphia, Pa.; London: Lippincott Williams & Wilkins.

Rubenson, D.L. and Runco, M.A. (1992). The economics of creativity & the psychology of economics: A rejoinder. *New Ideas in Psychology, 10*, 173–8.

Rubenson, D.L. and Runco, M.A. (1995). The Psychoeconomic View of Creative Work in Groups and Organizations. *Creativity and Innovation Management, 4*(4), 232–41.

Runco, M.A. (1996). Personal creativity: Definition and developmental issues. *New Directions for Child Development, 72*, 3–30.

Runco, M.A. (2004). Creativity. *Annu Rev Psychol, 55*, 657–87. doi: 10.1146/annurev.psych.55.090902.141502

Runco, M.A. (2005). Everyone Has Creative Potential. In R.J. Sternberg, E.L. Grigorenko and J.L. Singer (Eds), *Creativity: From potential to realization* (pp. 21–30). Washington, D.C.: American Psychological Association.

Runco, M.A. (2007a). *Creativity: Theories and themes: research, development and practice*. Amsterdam; London: Elsevier Academic Press.

Runco, M.A. (2007b). A hierarchial framwork for for the study of creativity. *New Horizons in Education, 55*, 1–9.

Runco, M.A. (2010). Divergent thinking, creativity & ideation. In J.C. Kaufman and R.J. Sternberg (Eds), *The Cambridge handbook of creativity* (pp. 413–46). Cambridge; New York: Cambridge University Press.

Runco, M.A. and Chand, I. (1994). Problem finding, evaluative thinking & creativity. In M.A. Runco (Ed.), *Problem finding, problem solving & creativity* (pp. 40–76). Norwood, N.J.: Ablex.

Runco, M.A. and Richards, R. (1997). *Eminent creativity, everyday creativity and health*. Greenwich, Conn.: Ablex Pub. Corp.

Runco, M.A. and Smith, W.R. (1992). Interpersonal and Intrapersonal Evaluations of Creative Ideas. *Personality and Individual Differences, 13*(3), 295–302. doi: Doi 10.1016/0191–8869(92)90105-X

Runco, M.A. and Vega, L. (1990). Evaluating the Creativity of Childrens Ideas. *Journal of Social Behavior and Personality, 5*(5), 439–452.

Runco, M.A., Mccarthy, K.A. and Svenson, E. (1994). Judgments of the Creativity of Artwork from Students and Professional Artists. *Journal of Psychology, 128*(1), 23–31.

Runco, M.A., Plucker, J.A. and Lim, W. (2000). Development and psychometric integrity of a measure of ideational behavior. *Creativity Research Journal, 13*(3–4), 393–400.

Runco, M.A., Noble, E.P., Reiter-Palmon, R., Acar, S., Ritchie, T. and Yurkovich, J.M. (2011). The genetic basis of creativity and ideational fluency. *Creativity Research Journal, 23*(4), 376–80.

Rybakowski, J.K. and Klonowska, P. (2011). Bipolar mood disorder, creativity and schizotypy: an experimental study. *Psychopathology, 44*(5), 296–302. doi: 10.1159/000322814

Sackett, D.L., Rosenberg, W.M., Gray, J.A., Haynes, R.B. and Richardson, W.S. (1996). Evidence based medicine: What it is and what it isn't. *BMJ, 312*(7023), 71–2.

Sadock, B.J., Sadock, V.A., Ruiz, P. and Kaplan, H.I. (2009). *Kaplan and Sadock's comprehensive textbook of psychiatry* (9th ed. / editors Benjamin J. Sadock, Virginia A. Sadock, Pedro Ruiz. ed.). Philadelphia, Pa.; London: Wolters Kluwer Health/Lippincott Williams & Wilkins.

Sanborn, K. (1886). *The vanity and insanity of genius.* New York: Coombes.

Santosa, C.M., Strong, C.M., Nowakowska, C., Wang, P.W., Rennicke, C.M. and Ketter, T.A. (2007). Enhanced creativity in bipolar disorder patients: A controlled study. *J Affect Disord, 100*(1–3), 31–9. doi: S0165–0327(06)00452–6 [pii] 10.1016/j.jad.2006.10.013

Sass, L.A. (2000a). Romanticism, creativity & the ambiguities of psychiatric diagnosis: Rejoinder to Kay Redfield Jamison. *Creativity Research Journal, 13*(1), 77–85.

Sass, L.A. (2000b). Schizophrenia, modernism & the 'creative imagination': On creativity and psychopathology. *Creativity Research Journal, 13*(1), 55–74.

Sawyer, R.K. (2010). Individual and Group Creativity. In J.C. Kaufman and R.J. Sternberg (Eds), *Cambridge handbooks in psychology* (pp. xvii, 489). Cambridge; New York: Cambridge University Press.

Sawyer, R.K. (2012a). Creativity and Mental Illness: Is There a Link?   Retrieved 27 April, 2014, from http://www.huffingtonpost.com/dr-r-keith-sawyer/creativity-and-mental-ill_b_2059806.html

Sawyer, R.K. (2012b). *Explaining creativity: The science of human innovation* (2nd ed.). New York: Oxford University Press.

Schafer, G., Feilding, A., Morgan, C.J., Agathangelou, M., Freeman, T.P. and Valerie Curran, H. (2012). Investigating the interaction between schizotypy, divergent thinking and cannabis use. *Conscious Cogn, 21*(1), 292–8. doi: 10.1016/j.concog.2011.11.009

Schatzberg, A.F. and Nemeroff, C.B. (2009). *The American Psychiatric Publishing textbook of psychopharmacology* (4th ed.). Washington, D.C.: American Psychiatric Pub.

Schlesinger, J. (2004). Creativity and mental health. *Br J Psychiatry, 184*, 184; author reply 184–5.

Schlesinger, J. (2009). Creative Mythconceptions: A Closer Look at the Evidence for the 'Mad Genius' Hypothesis. *Psychology of Aesthetics Creativity and the Arts, 3*(2), 62–72. doi: 10.1037/A0013975

Schlesinger, J. (2012). *The insanity hoax: Exposing the myth of the mad genius.* Ardsley-on-Hudson, N.Y.: Shrinktunes Media.

Schlesinger, J. (2014). Building Connections on Sand: The Cautionary Chapter. In J.C. Kaufman (Ed.), *Creativity and mental illness* (in press).

Schmechel, D.E. (2007). Art, alpha-1-antitrypsin polymorphisms and intense creative energy: blessing or curse? *Neurotoxicology, 28*(5), 899–914. doi: 10.1016/j. neuro.2007.05.011

Schmechel, D.E. and Edwards, C.L. (2012). Fibromyalgia, mood disorders & intense creative energy: A1AT polymorphisms are not always silent. *Neurotoxicology, 33*(6), 1454–72. doi: 10.1016/j.neuro.2012.03.001

Schmithorst, V.J., Wilke, M., Dardzinski, B.J. and Holland, S.K. (2005). Cognitive functions correlate with white matter architecture in a normal pediatric population: A diffusion tensor MRI study. *Hum Brain Mapp, 26*(2), 139–47. doi: 10.1002/hbm.20149

Schou, M. (1979). Artistic productivity and lithium prophylaxis in manic-depressive illness. *Br J Psychiatry, 135*, 97–103.

Schou, M., Thomsen, K. and Armitage, P. (1971). Prophylactic Lithium. *The Lancet, 297*(7708), 1066.

Schuldberg, D. (2005). Eysenck Personality Questionnaire scales and paper-and-pencil tests related to creativity. *Psychol Rep, 97*(1), 180–2.

Schuldberg, D., French, C., Stone, B.L. and Heberle, J. (1988). Creativity and schizotypal traits. Creativity test scores and perceptual aberration, magical ideation & impulsive nonconformity. *J Nerv Ment Dis, 176*(11), 648–57.

Senn, S. (2011). Francis Galton and regression to the mean. *Significance, 8*(3), 124–6. doi: 10.1111/j.1740-9713.2011.00509.x

Sharma, M., Krüger, R. and Gasser, T. (2014). From genome-wide association studies to next-generation sequencing: Lessons from the past and planning for the future. *JAMA Neurology, 71*(1), 5–6. doi: 10.1001/jamaneurol.2013.3682

Shaw, E.D., Mann, J.J., Stokes, P.E. and Manevitz, A.Z. (1986). Effects of lithium carbonate on associative productivity and idiosyncrasy in bipolar outpatients. *Am J Psychiatry, 143*(9), 1166–9.

Shaw, J., Claridge, G. and Clark, K. (2001). Schizotypy and the shift from dextrality: A study of handedness in a large non-clinical sample. *Schizophr Res, 50*(3), 181–9.

Shorter, E. (1997). *A history of psychiatry: From the era of the asylum to the age of Prozac.* New York: John Wiley & Sons.

Sieborger, F.T., Ferstl, E.C. and von Cramon, D.Y. (2007). Making sense of nonsense: an fMRI study of task induced inference processes during discourse comprehension. *Brain Res, 1166*, 77–91. doi: S0006-8993(07)01167-5 [pii] 10.1016/j.brainres.2007.05.079

Sigg, J.M. and Gargiulo, R.M. (1980). Creativity and cognitive style in learning disabled and nondisabled school age children. *Psychol Rep, 46*(1), 299–305.

Silvia, P.J. and Kaufman, J.C. (2010). Creativity and mental illness. In J.C. Kaufman and R.J. Sternberg (Eds), *The Cambridge handbook of creativity.* Cambridge: Cambridge University Press.

Silvia, P.J. and Kimbrel, N.A. (2010). A Dimensional Analysis of Creativity and Mental Illness: Do Anxiety and Depression Symptoms Predict Creative Cognition, Creative Accomplishments & Creative Self-Concepts? *Psychology of Aesthetics Creativity and the Arts, 4*(1), 2–10. doi: Doi 10.1037/A0016494

Simeonova, D.I., Chang, K.D., Strong, C. and Ketter, T.A. (2005). Creativity in familial bipolar disorder. *J Psychiatr Res, 39*(6), 623–31. doi: S0022-3956(05)00009-9 [pii] 10.1016/j.jpsychires.2005.01.005

Simon, H. (1988). Creativity and motivation: A response to Csikszentmihalyi. *New Ideas in Psychology, 6*, 177–81.

Simon, H.A. and Chase, W.G. (1973). Skill in Chess. *American Scientist, 61*(4), 394–403.

Simonton, D.K. (1977a). Creative Productivity, Age & Stress – Biographical Time-Series Analysis of 10 Classical Composers. *Journal of Personality and Social Psychology, 35*(11), 791–804. doi: 10.1037//0022–3514.35.11.791

Simonton, D.K. (1977b). Eminence, Creativity & Geographic Marginality – Recursive Structural Equation Model. *Journal of Personality and Social Psychology, 35*(11), 805–16. doi: 10.1037//0022–3514.35.11.805

Simonton, D.K. (1984a). *Genius, creativity & leadership: Historiometric inquiries*. Cambridge, Mass.: Harvard University Press.

Simonton, D.K. (1984b). Is the Marginality Effect All That Marginal. *Social Studies of Science, 14*(4), 621–2. doi: 10.1177/030631284014004005

Simonton, D.K. (1985). Quality, Quantity & Age – the Careers of Ten Distinguished Psychologists. *International Journal of Aging and Human Development, 21*(4), 241–54. doi: 10.2190/Kb7e-A45m-X8x7-Dqj4

Simonton, D.K. (1988a). Age and Outstanding Achievement: What Do We Know After a Century of Research? *Psychological Bulletin, 104*(2), 251–67.

Simonton, D.K. (1988b). *Scientific genius: A psychology of science*. Cambridge; New York: Cambridge University Press.

Simonton, D.K. (1991a). Career Landmarks in Science – Individual-Differences and Interdisciplinary Contrasts. *Developmental Psychology, 27*(1), 119–30. doi: 10.1037//0012–1649.27.1.119

Simonton, D.K. (1991b). Emergence and Realization of Genius – the Lives and Works of 120 Classical Composers. *Journal of Personality and Social Psychology, 61*(5), 829–40. doi: 10.1037/0022–3514.61.5.829

Simonton, D.K. (1997). Creative productivity: A predictive and explanatory model of career trajectories and landmarks. *Psychological Review, 104*(1), 66–89. doi: 10.1037/0033–295x.104.1.66

Simonton, D.K. (1998). Fickle fashion versus immortal fame: Transhistorical assessments of creative products in the opera house. *Journal of Personality and Social Psychology, 75*(1), 198–210. doi: 10.1037/0022–3514.75.1.198

Simonton, D.K. (1999a). Creativity as blind variation and selective retention: Is the creative process Darwinian? *Psychological Inquiry, 10*(4), 309–28.

Simonton, D.K. (1999b). *Origins of genius: Darwinian perspectives on creativity*. New York; Oxford: Oxford University Press.

Simonton, D.K. (2000). Creative development as acquired expertise: Theoretical issues and an empirical test. *Developmental Review, 20*(2), 283–318. doi: 10.1006/drev.1999.0504

Simonton, D.K. (2003). Scientific creativity as constrained stochastic behavior: The integration of product, person & process perspectives. *Psychological Bulletin, 129*, 475–94.

Simonton, D.K. (2006). *Creative genius, knowledge & reason: The lives and works of eminent creators*. Cambridge: Cambridge University Press.

Simonton, D.K. (2012). Quantifying creativity: can measures span the spectrum? *Dialogues Clin Neurosci, 14*(1), 100–4.

Sitton, S.C. and Hughes, R.B. (1995). Creativity, depression & circannual variation. *Psychol Rep, 77*(3 Pt 1), 907–10.

Smith, C.A.B. (1997). Galton, Francis *Leading Personalities in Statistical Sciences* (pp. 109–11): John Wiley & Sons, Inc.

Smith, G.J. and Carlsson, I. (1983). Creativity and anxiety: An experimental study. *Scand J Psychol, 24*(2), 107–15.

Socialstyrelsen (National Board of Health and Welfare in Sweden). (2010). *Internationell statistisk klassifikation av sjukdomar och relaterade hälsoproblem – systematisk förteckning (ICD-10-SE) (Swedish Verison of International Statistical Classification of Diseases and Related Health Problems, Tenth Revision (ICD-10)* Retrieved from http://www.socialstyrelsen.se/publikationer2010/2010–11–13.

Soderqvist, T. (1994). Darwinian Overtones – Jerne, Niels,K. and the Origin of the Selection Theory of Antibody-Formation. *Journal of the History of Biology, 27*(3), 481–529. doi: 10.1007/Bf01058995

Soeiro-de-Souza, M.G., Dias, V.V., Bio, D.S., Post, R.M. and Moreno, R.A. (2011). Creativity and executive function across manic, mixed and depressive episodes in bipolar I disorder. *J Affect Disord, 135*(1–3), 292–7. doi: 10.1016/j.jad.2011.06.024

Soeiro-de-Souza, M.G., Post, R.M., de Sousa, M.L., Missio, G., do Prado, C.M., Gattaz, W.F., ... Machado-Vieira, R. (2012). Does BDNF genotype influence creative output in bipolar I manic patients? *Journal of Affective Disorders, 139*(2), 181–6. doi: 10.1016/j.jad.2012.01.036

Sperry, R.W. (1964). The Great Cerebral Commissure. *Sci Am, 210*, 42–52.

Spieth, H.T. (1974). Courtship behavior in Drosophila. *Annu Rev Entomol, 19*, 385–405. doi: 10.1146/annurev.en.19.010174.002125

Srivastava, S., Childers, M.E., Baek, J.H., Strong, C.M., Hill, S.J., Warsett, K.S., ... Ketter, T.A. (2010). Toward interaction of affective and cognitive contributors to creativity in bipolar disorders: A controlled study. *J Affect Disord, 125*(1–3), 27–34. doi: 10.1016/j.jad.2009.12.018

Stack, S. (1996). Gender and suicide risk among artists: A multivariate analysis. *Suicide Life Threat Behav, 26*(4), 374–9.

Stanghellini, G. and Rosfort, R. (2010). Affective temperament and personal identity. *J Affect Disord, 126*(1–2), 317–20. doi: 10.1016/j.jad.2010.02.129

Starchenko, M.G., Bekhtereva, N.P., Pakhomov, S.V. and Medvedev, S.V. (2003). Study of the brain organization of creative thinking. *Human Physiology, 29*(5), 652–3.

Stein, E. and Lipton, P. (1989). Where Guesses Come from – Evolutionary Epistemology and the Anomaly of Guided Variation. *Biology and Philosophy, 4*(1), 33–56. doi: 10.1007/Bf00144038

Stein, M.I. (1953). Creativity and culture. *Journal of Psychology, 36*, 311–22.

Stern, T.A. (2008). *Massachusetts General Hospital comprehensive clinical psychiatry* (1st ed.). Philadelphia, Pa.: Mosby/Elsevier.

Sternberg, R.J. and Davidson, J.E. (1995). *The nature of insight*. Cambridge, Mass.: MIT Press.

Stohs, J.H. (1992). Intrinsic motivation and sustained art activity among male fine and applied artists. *Creativity Research Journal, 5*(3), 245–52.

Stoltenberg, S.F. (1997). Coming to terms with heritability. *Genetica, 99*(2–3), 89–96.

Strong, C.M., Nowakowska, C., Santosa, C.M., Wang, P.W., Kraemer, H.C. and Ketter, T.A. (2007). Temperament-creativity relationships in mood disorder patients, healthy controls and highly creative individuals. *J Affect Disord, 100*(1–3), 41–8. doi: S0165–0327(06)00454-X [pii] 10.1016/j.jad.2006.10.015

Stulp, G., Buunk, A.P., Pollet, T.V., Nettle, D. and Verhulst, S. (2013). Are Human Mating Preferences with Respect to Height Reflected in Actual Pairings? *PLoS One, 8*(1), e54186. doi: 10.1371/journal.pone.0054186

Sully, J. (1884). *Outlines of Psychology, with special reference to the theory of education.* London: Longmans & Co.

Sun, J., Kuo, P.H., Riley, B.P., Kendler, K.S. and Zhao, Z. (2008). Candidate genes for schizophrenia: a survey of association studies and gene ranking. *Am J Med Genet B Neuropsychiatr Genet, 147B*(7), 1173–81. doi: 10.1002/ajmg.b.30743

Symonds, R.L. and Williams, P. (1976). Seasonal variation in the incidence of mania. *Br J Psychiatry, 129*, 45–8.

Synder, A., Mulcahy, E., Taylor, J., Mitchell, D.J., Sachdev, P. and Gandevia, S.C. (2003). Savant-like skills exposed in normal people by suppressing the left fronto-temporal lobe. *Journal of Integrative Neuroscience, 2*, 149–58.

Thys, E., Sabbe, B. and De Hert, M. (2014a). The assessment of creativity in creativity/psychopathology research – a systematic review. *Cogn Neuropsychiatry.* doi: 10.1080/13546805.2013.877384

Thys, E., Sabbe, B. and De Hert, M. (2014b). Creativity and Psychopathology: A Systematic Review. *Psychopathology.* doi: 10.1159/000357822

Tonelli, G. (1973). Genius from the Renaissance to 1770. In P.P. Wiener (Ed.), *Dictionary of the history of ideas* (pp. 293–7). New York: Scribner.

Torrance, E.P. (1982). Hemisphericity and creative functioning. *Journal of Research and Development in Education, 15*, 29–37.

Torrance, E.P. and Ball, O.E. (1984). *Torrance tests of creative thinking: Streamlined administration and scoring manual* (Revised ed.). Bensonville, Ill.: Scholastic Testing Service.

Tremblay, C.H., Grosskopf, S. and Yang, K. (2010). Brainstorm: Occupational choice, bipolar illness and creativity. *Econ Hum Biol, 8*(2), 233–41. doi: S1570–677X (10)00002-X [pii] 10.1016/j.ehb.2010.01.001

Tucker, P.K., Rothwell, S.J., Armstrong, M.S. and McConaghy, N. (1982). Creativity, divergent and allusive thinking in students and visual artists. *Psychol Med, 12*(4), 835–41.

Turner, M.A. (1999). Generating novel ideas: Fluency performance in high-functioning and learning disabled individuals with autism. *J Child Psychol Psychiatry, 40*(2), 189–201.

Ukkola-Vuoti, L., Kanduri, C., Oikkonen, J., Buck, G., Blancher, C., Raijas, P., ... Jarvela, I. (2013). Genome-wide copy number variation analysis in extended families and unrelated individuals characterized for musical aptitude and creativity in music. *PLoS One, 8*(2), e56356. doi: 10.1371/journal.pone. 0056356

Ukkola, L.T., Onkamo, P., Raijas, P., Karma, K. and Jarvela, I. (2009). Musical aptitude is associated with AVPR1A-haplotypes. *PLoS One, 4*(5), e5534. doi: 10.1371/journal.pone.0005534

Van Schouwenburg, M., Aarts, E. and Cools, R. (2010). Dopaminergic modulation of cognitive control: Distinct roles for the prefrontal cortex and the basal ganglia. *Curr Pharm Des, 16*(18), 2026–32.

Vandenberg, S.G. (1967). Hereditary factors in psychological variables in man, with a special emphasis on cognition. In J.N. Spuhler (Ed.), *Genetic diversity and human behavior* (pp. 99–134). Chicago: Aldine.

Vellante, M., Zucca, G., Preti, A., Sisti, D., Rocchi, M.B., Akiskal, K.K. and Akiskal, H.S. (2011). Creativity and affective temperaments in non-clinical professional artists: an empirical psychometric investigation. *J Affect Disord, 135*(1–3), 28–36. doi: 10.1016/j.jad.2011.06.062

Visscher, P.M., Hill, W.G. and Wray, N.R. (2008). Heritability in the genomics era – concepts and misconceptions. *Nature reviews. Genetics, 9*(4), 255–66. doi: 10.1038/nrg2322

Visscher, P.M., Medland, S.E., Ferreira, M.A., Morley, K.I., Zhu, G., Cornes, B.K., ... Martin, N.G. (2006). Assumption-free estimation of heritability from genome-wide identity-by-descent sharing between full siblings. *PLoS genetics, 2*(3), e41. doi: 10.1371/journal.pgen.0020041

Vygotsky, L.S. (2004). Imagination and Creativity in Childhood. *Journal of Russian and East European Psychology, 42*, 7–97.

Wallach, M.A. (1980). Citation Classic – Modes of Thinking in Young-Children – Study of the Creativity-Intelligence Distinction. *Current Contents/Social and Behavioral Sciences* (13), 14–14.

Wallach, M.A. and Kogan, N. (1965). *Modes of thinking in young children.* New York: Holt, Rinehart & Winston.

Wallach, M.A. and Wing, C. (1969). *The talented student.* New York: Holt, Rinehart & Winston.

Wallas, G. (1926). *Art of Thought.* London: Jonathan Cape.

Waller, N.G., Bouchard, T.J., Lykken, D.T. and Tellegen, A. (1993). Creativity, heritability, familiality: Which word does not belong? *Psychological Inquiry, 4*(3), 235–7.

Wang, J., Conder, J.A., Blitzer, D.N. and Shinkareva, S.V. (2010). Neural representation of abstract and concrete concepts: A meta-analysis of neuroimaging studies. *Hum Brain Mapp.* doi: 10.1002/hbm.20950

Wei, M.H. (2011). The social adjustment, academic performance & creativity of Taiwanese children with Tourette's syndrome. *Psychol Rep, 108*(3), 791–8.

Weinstein, S. and Graves, R.E. (2002). Are creativity and schizotypy products of a right hemisphere bias? *Brain Cogn, 49*(1), 138–51. doi: 10.1006/brcg.2001.1493

Weisberg, R.W. (1994). Genius and Madness – a Quasi-Experimental Test of the Hypothesis that Manic-Depression Increases Creativity. *Psychological Science, 5*(6), 361–7.

Welling, H. (2007). Four Mental Operations in Creative Cognition: The Importance of Abstraction. *Creativity Research Journal, 19*(2–3), 163–77.

White, H.A. and Shah, P. (2006). Uninhibited imaginations: Creativity in adults with Attention-Deficit/Hyperactivity Disorder. *Personality and Individual Differences, 40*(6), 1121–31. doi: 10.1016/j.paid.2005.11.007

White, H.A. and Shah, P. (2011). Creative style and achievement in adults with attention-deficit/hyperactivity disorder. *Personality and Individual Differences, 50*(5), 673–7. doi: DOI 10.1016/j.paid.2010.12.015

Wills, G.I. (2003). Forty lives in the bebop business: Mental health in a group of eminent jazz musicians. *Br J Psychiatry, 183*, 255–9.

Witt, L.A. and Beorkrem, M. (1989). Climate for creative productivity as a predictor of research usefulness and organizational effectiveness in an RandD organization. *Creativity Research Journal, 2*, 30–40.

Wittkower, R. and Wittkower, M. (2007). *Born under Saturn: the character and conduct of artists: a documented history from antiquity to the French Revolution.* New York: New York Review Books.

World Health Organization. (1967). *International Classification of Diseases, Eight Revision (ICD-8).* Geneva, Switzerland: World Health Organization.

World Health Organization. (1977). *International Classification of Diseases, Ninth Revision (ICD-9)*. Geneva, Switzerland: World Health Organization.

World Health Organization. (1993). *The ICD-10 Classification of Mental and Behavioural Disorders Diagnostic criteria for research*. Geneva, Switzerland: World Health Organization.

World Health Organization. (2004). *International Statistical Classification of Diseases and Related Health Problems, 10th Revision (ICD-10)* (2 ed.). Geneva, Switzerland: World Health Organization.

Young, L.N., Winner, E. and Cordes, S. (2013). Heightened Incidence of Depressive Symptoms in Adolescents Involved in the Arts. *Psychology of Aesthetics Creativity and the Arts, 7*(2), 197–202. doi: 10.1037/a0030468

Zehavi, A. and Zahavi, A. (1997). *The handicap principle: A missing piece of Darwin's puzzle*. New York: Oxford University Press.

Zilsel, E. (1926). *Die enstehung des geniebegriffes* [*The origin of the genius concept*]. Tübingen: Mohr.

Index

Page numbers in *italics* refer to tables and figures.

CPSIA information can be obtained
at www.ICGtesting.com
Printed in the USA
LVOW10*2309081117
555580LV00005B/39/P